WALKING
San Francisco

A Step-by-Step Tour of the City by the Bay

Second Edition

LIZ GANS & RICK NEWBY
REVISED BY TRACY SALCEDO-CHOURRÉ

FALCONGUIDES

GUILFORD, CONNECTICUT
HELENA, MONTANA

AN IMPRINT OF ROWMAN & LITTLEFIELD

*For Marg and Joe, who have walked San
Francisco for more than fifty years*

*In memoriam
Elaine Isabelle Crowe Newby (1925–1998)*

*For my amazing mother, Judy Salcedo, a
fifth-generation San Franciscan*

FALCONGUIDES®

FalconGuides is an imprint of Rowman & Littlefield

Falcon, FalconGuides, and Outfit Your Mind are registered trademarks of Rowman & Littlefield.

Copyright © 2014 by Rowman & Littlefield

British Library Cataloguing-in-Publication Information available

Library of Congress Cataloging-in-Publication Data available

ISBN 978-0-7627-9600-7 (paperback)

∞™ The paper used in this publication meets the minimum requirements of American National Standard for Information Sciences—Permanence of Paper for Printed Library Materials, ANSI/NISO Z39.48-1992.

Contents

Parklands

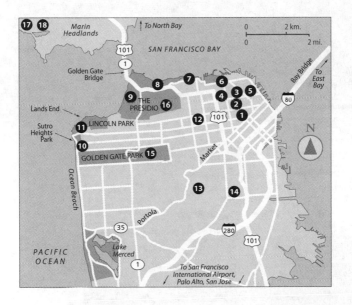

Marin
Headlands

To North Bay

SAN FRANCISCO BAY

0   2 km.

0   2 mi.

Bay Bridge

To East Bay

Golden Gate
Bridge

Lands End

THE PRESIDIO

Sutro
Heights
Park

LINCOLN PARK

GOLDEN GATE PARK

Market

Portola

Ocean Beach

PACIFIC
OCEAN

Lake
Merced

To San Francisco
International Airport,
Palo Alto, San Jose

N

Map Legend

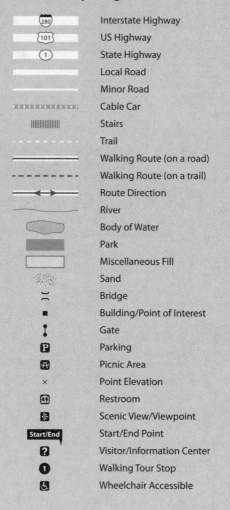

280	Interstate Highway
101	US Highway
1	State Highway
	Local Road
	Minor Road
	Cable Car
	Stairs
	Trail
	Walking Route (on a road)
	Walking Route (on a trail)
← →	Route Direction
	River
	Body of Water
	Park
	Miscellaneous Fill
	Sand
≍	Bridge
■	Building/Point of Interest
	Gate
P	Parking
🛱	Picnic Area
×	Point Elevation
🚻	Restroom
🔍	Scenic View/Viewpoint
Start/End	Start/End Point
?	Visitor/Information Center
1	Walking Tour Stop
♿	Wheelchair Accessible

Foreword

It has been the mission of FalconGuides to help millions of people enjoy America's wild outside, showing them where to paddle, hike, bike, bird, fish, climb, and drive. With this walking series, Falcon invites you to experience the country from its sidewalks; to stroll through some of America's most interesting and beautiful cities.

It's no big secret that historic and scenic treasures abide within cities, but sometimes the beauty of the urban landscape is overlooked. While nothing can replace the serenity and inspiration of the backcountry, cityscapes can inspire similar awe. The steel and glass of municipal mountains reflect sunlight, create canyons, and make walkers feel small. Birds sing in city parks, water burbles in fountains, and abundant wildlife crowds the sidewalks—fellow human beings.

Falcon's outdoor guidebooks encourage readers not only to explore and enjoy America's natural beauty but also to preserve and protect it. Likewise, our cities should be enjoyed and explored, and their irreplaceable treasures cared for and preserved. The desire to be a caretaker may germinate by developing intimate knowledge of a place, and taking a long walk in a new neighborhood may be the first step in firing up that desire.

When travelers and walkers want to explore something inspirational and beautiful, we hope they will lace up their walking shoes and wander through one of this country's many cities. For there, along the walkways, they are sure to discover the excitement, history, beauty, and charm of urban America.

—*The Editors*

Acknowledgments

First, and most of all, we want to thank Margaret and Joe Gans, who encouraged, nurtured, and walked with us while we wrote *Walking San Francisco*. Their home on Telegraph Hill was our San Francisco haven, and their enthusiasm for this project was boundless.

We want to thank the wonderful Bay Area friends and acquaintances who took us into their homes, gave us hot tips for good restaurants, intriguing attractions, and great walks—and sometimes tested the walks for us: Richard Gans; Peter Merts; Michele Foyer and Mark Fredenburg; Peter Rutledge Koch; Harold Charns and Rose Schubert; John Palmer and Leslie Cobb; Gilda and Gregory Loew; Linda Maki and Doug, Nathan, and Aaron Groom; Bob Hoover; Anne Appleby and Melissa Kwasny; Ed Gilbert; Griff and Chris Williams; Gary and Karen Carson; Paul and Sandra Tsang; and John and Trish Kinsella.

We owe a special debt to Jennifer Thompson. Thanks to J. M. Cooper and Peter Merts for invaluable photographic advice, and to Adolph Gasser Inc., Third Eye Photographics, and Jeff Van Tine for their darkroom magic.

Julie Soller, public relations coordinator at the San Francisco Travel Association, gave us helpful guidance, as did Kathleen Mozena of the bureau's membership office. Paul McBride of Wheelchairs of Berkeley graciously helped us decide which walks are wheelchair accessible. Anita Hill, executive director of Yerba Buena Alliance, kept us up-to-date on developments in Yerba Buena Gardens. Bob Yeargin of City Guides pointed out many of the sights we mention in our Chinatown walk; and Patricia Rose of the Precita Eyes Mural Arts Center showed us the Mission's rich mural heritage. In Ina Coolbrith Park, Charles the Thinker offered spiritual advice and several walk ideas. And Jeanne Fidler told us much about the bird life of the Marin Headlands.

We want to also offer our gratitude to the many folks at the Golden Gate National Recreation Area (GGNRA) who unstintingly provided guidance about particular walks in the GGNRA. They include Dean J. Whittaker, Bob G. Holloway, J. Sherman, and Cathy Petrick and Diana Roberts. Carol Prince of the Golden Gate National Parks Association guided us through the changes under way along the Golden Gate Promenade. And special thanks to Chris Powell of the GGNRA, who oversaw the review of all walks within the park, and to John Cunnane, supervisory park ranger at the San Francisco Maritime National Historical Park, who reviewed our Fisherman's Wharf walk.

Our editor, Judith Galas, was a consummate professional throughout, and her clear and savvy direction made the research and writing of *Walking San Francisco* a real joy. Gayle Shirley, our editor at Falcon Publishing, provided great advice and was infinitely patient. Finally, our gratitude to Randall Green, former Falcon guidebook editor, who signed us up for this project, and to Bill Schneider and Chris Cauble, who made it happen.

—Liz Gans and Rick Newby

For the revised edition, I'd like to thank the original authors for selecting wonderful walks and conducting thorough research. The foundation of this guide remains virtually intact; I have added extensions and modifications to a few of the routes and updated all contact and access information. It's tough to improve on a good thing. San

Francisco is home turf, but with Liz and Rick's guidance, I discovered new places, revisited old favorites, and learned more about the city's rich natural and cultural history.

Thanks to Alison Reimers, Patrice Fusillo, JT Long, Mike Dodd, Linda Dehzad, Dave Macon, Jennifer Losin Decker, Marina Zachau (I didn't tell anybody), Denise Santa Cruz-Bohman, and Audra Bodwell for their advice on places to eat. Kerin McTaggart and Karen Charland entertained me on my walks (gotta love cell phones). Thanks to my mom and dad, Judy and Jesse Salcedo, along with the generations of Blakistons, Hammertons, and Schombergs, I can say I am not only a native San Franciscan, but also a sixth-generation San Franciscan. Many thanks to Laurie Armstrong of San Francisco Travel, Susan Cervantes of Precita Eyes Muralists, and James Marks of the Golden Gate National Recreation Area for their review of the revised manuscript. I am forever grateful to the wonderful crew that pulls together FalconGuides for Rowman & Littlefield. Their experience, patience, and encouragement is priceless and has sustained me through many a guidebook-compilation adventure.

And, as always, thanks to my inspirational sons, Penn, Cruz, and Jesse.

—Tracy Salcedo-Chourré

Introduction: Come Walk San Francisco

Mythical San Francisco, fabled for its gorgeous natural setting, its cable cars, its earthquakes, its status at the forefront of cultural innovation, and the charm of its distinctive neighborhoods. Mild in climate and quirky in character, the city overflows with history, attractions, and distinctive neighborhoods to explore. For the walker, the city offers breathtaking vistas and challenging topography, its steep hills laced with storied Victorians and staircases lined with gardens. The city is compact: An ambitious pedestrian can see much of it in a single day, traversing a startling array of cultural enclaves and encountering microclimates that range from bone-chilling to tropical. And the hungry walker has hit the jackpot—San Francisco is a culinary mecca, boasting more than 3,000 restaurants, many of them world-class.

In addition to a network of city parks—including the wonderland that is Golden Gate Park—San Francisco is at the heart of the spectacular and diverse Golden Gate National Recreation Area (GGNRA). One of the largest urban national parks in the world, the GGNRA stretches beyond city limits to encompass Alcatraz Island, the Marin Headlands and Muir Woods National Monument north of the Golden Gate, and south onto Sweeney Ridge, where Spanish explorer Gaspar de Portola first laid eyes on San Francisco Bay. The park also protects some of the city's most beloved landmarks, from the Cliff House to Fort Point. In addition, it wraps around the Presidio of San Francisco, composed as much of historical sites as of wildland, and supported by an innovative private-public partnership.

Walking San Francisco takes full advantage of the GGNRA, featuring eight walks within the recreation

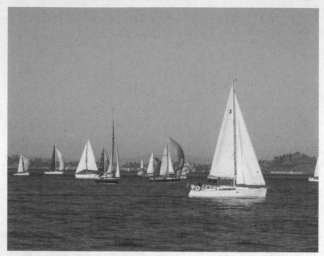

Walkers must stick to dry land, but they can enjoy the spectacle of sailboats on San Francisco Bay.

area's boundaries. These walks stand in contrast to those inside the city itself. Imagine: One day you're jostling down vibrant, crowded Fisherman's Wharf, and the next you find relative seclusion winding down a forested trail in the Presidio. One day you flow with the crowds in Chinatown or take in the vibrant murals of the Mission District, and the next you trace the edge of the continent on the Coastal Trail at Lands End. You can spend a morning on the Golden Gate Promenade, watching the fog roll back through the Golden Gate, and then pass the afternoon on steep streets below Twin Peaks, checking out some of the city's most photogenic Victorian architecture.

Walking the streets and boulevards of San Francisco will give you a feel for its pulse and personality. From its sidewalks you can appreciate its architecture and venture into quaint shops, local museums, and great eateries. From its nature paths you can smell the flowers, glimpse the wildlife, gaze at a lake, or watch the surf crash onto the sand. Only by walking can you get close enough to read historical plaques. Only by walking can you mingle with the people: vendors, families, old-timers, couples holding hands. When you walk the city, you get it all—adventure, scenery, local color, good exercise, and fun.

San Francisco has been called the loveliest city on earth. Discover this truth for yourself. Try *Walking San Francisco*.

How to Use This Guide

This book is designed so that you can easily find the walks that match your interests, time, and energy level. Begin by checking out the Trip Planner. This table will give you the basic information you'll need to decide on a walk: its distance, estimated walking time, and relative difficulty. The pictures or icons in the table tell you specific things about the walk:

📷 The route will appeal to the shutterbug. Bring your camera: You will have great views of the city or the surrounding landscapes and are likely to get some wonderful scenic shots.

✕ Food and/or beverages are available somewhere along the route. Walks that do not have the food icon probably are along nature trails or in noncommercial areas of the city.

🛒 You'll have a chance to shop along the route. Descriptions of the types of stores you will find are in the walk descriptions.

👫 Kids will enjoy something specific along this route—a park, zoo, museum, or play equipment. In most cases walks with this icon are short and follow an easy, fairly level path. You know your young walking companions best. If your children are patient and do not tire easily, you can choose longer, harder walks. In fact, depending on a child's age and energy, all of the walks in this book are possible.

🏢 Your path will take you primarily through urban areas, passing along paved routes among buildings and small city parks.

🍃 The route leads through a large park or natural setting where you will enjoy a wilder landscape.

♿ The wheelchair icon means the path is accessible. The route is easy for someone pushing a wheelchair or stroller, meaning it is mostly or entirely paved, curb cuts or ramps have been installed along the entire route, and you'll find a wheelchair-accessible restroom along the way. If you use a wheelchair and can negotiate curbs and dirt paths, or have the ability to wheel for longer distances and on uneven surfaces, you may want to skim the walks that do not carry this symbol, as you may enjoy them as well. If in doubt, call the contact source for guidance.

Walk Descriptions

At the start of each walk description, you will find specific information describing the route and what you can expect on your walk:

General location: The walk's general location within the city or within a specific area of the city.

Special attractions: If the walk has museums, historic homes, restaurants, or wildlife-viewing opportunities, it will be noted here.

Difficulty: An ordinary person in reasonable health can complete the walks selected for this book. A walk with a moderate rating can be completed by an "average" walker, but that walker may feel tired or sore when he or she has completed the route. How easy or hard a walk may be depends on each person's level of fitness. Here are general guidelines as to what the difficulty ratings indicate:

A walk rated **easy** is generally flat, with few or no hills. Most likely you will be walking on a maintained surface of concrete, asphalt, wood, or packed earth. The path is easy to follow, and you will be only a block or so from a phone, other people, or businesses. If the walk is less than a mile, you may be able to walk comfortably in street shoes.

A **moderate** walk includes some hills; a few may be quite steep. The route may include stretches of sand, dirt, gravel, or crushed rock. You should wear good walking shoes.

A walk rated **strenuous** is likely along an unpaved path peppered with rocks, tree roots, and patches of vegetation. The trail may have steep ups and downs, and you may have to pause now and then to interpret walking directions against the natural setting. Carrying water is advisable, and you may be alone or secluded for long stretches.

Walks with this rating also include those with long uphill stretches or staircases. Walking shoes are a must, and hiking boots may be helpful.

Distance: Mileages for each walk were verified with a GPS unit. The mileage you log may differ depending on detours you may choose to take. San Francisco's street grid is fairly straightforward, so you can shorten or lengthen routes without too much difficulty.

Estimated time: The time allotted for each route is based on walking time only, which has been calculated at about 30 minutes per mile—a slow pace. Most people have no trouble walking a mile in half an hour, and people with walking experience often walk a 20-minute mile. You'll go slower when on steep hills and negotiating staircases. If the walk includes museums, shops, or restaurants, you may want to add sightseeing time to the estimate.

Services: If restrooms, parking, refreshments, or information centers are available, you'll find them, along with their general locations, listed here.

Restrictions: The restriction most often noted is whether the route is suitable for pets—primarily dogs, which must be leashed in the city. San Francisco also has a strict "pooper-scooper" law. Dogs are allowed to run leash-free in areas of the GGNRA, but those rules are under perpetual review; contact the park to find out where your dog can run free. The "Restrictions" entry may also include the hours or days a museum or business is open, age requirements, or whether you can ride a bike on the path. If there is something you cannot do on this walk, it will be noted.

For more information: Each walk includes at least one contact source for more information. If an agency

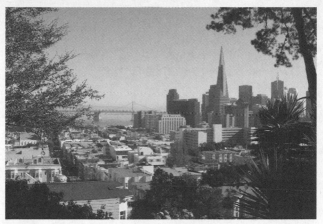

The Bay Bridge and Transamerica Pyramid as seen from the Greenwich Street stairs on Telegraph Hill.

or business is named as a contact, its phone number and address are also included in appendix B.

Getting started: This entry includes specific directions to the starting point. All of these walks are closed loops or out-and-back routes, which means they begin and end at the same point. Provided you are able to park nearby, or that you arrived at the starting point via public transit, you do not have to worry about finding your car or your way back to the bus stop when your walk is over.

Some walks can be started at any point in a given location—for example, at any corner of Union Square. The directions begin at a specific starting point, but this section will tell you if it is possible to pick up the walk at other locations. If you are staying at a downtown hotel, it is likely that a walk passes in front of or near your hotel's entrance.

Public transportation: San Francisco has an excellent public transportation system. If it is possible to take a bus or commuter train to the walk's starting point, you will find that noted. You may also find information about where the bus or train stops.

Overview: Every part of the city has a story. This section includes the story of the people, neighborhood, and/or history connected to the walk.

The Walk: In this section you will find specific and detailed directions, as well as learn more about the sights you pass. Those who want only the directions and none of the extras can find the straightforward information here.

For Your Comfort and Safety

What to Wear

The best advice for walking in San Francisco is to wear comfortable clothing and bring layers. Leave behind anything that binds, pinches, rides up, falls down, slips off the shoulder, or comes undone. The weather in the city can change from mile to mile, and the fog can roll in with surprising quickness, so carrying a sweatshirt or light jacket is always recommended.

What to Take

Always carry water. Strap a bottle to your fanny pack or tuck a bottle in a pocket. If you are walking several miles with a dog, bring along a small bowl so your pet can have a drink, too. Carry some water even if you will be walking where refreshments are available. Taking small sips throughout a walk is a more effective way to stay hydrated than taking one large drink at the walk's end. Avoid drinks with caffeine or alcohol because they deplete rather than replenish your body.

Trip Planner			
Walk	Difficulty	Distance (miles)	Time (hours)
Heart of the City			
1. Downtown	Easy	3.3	2
2. Chinatown	Easy	1.8	1
3. North Beach and Coit Tower	Strenuous	2.3	1.5
4. Russian Hill	Strenuous	3.9	2.5
Along the Bay			
5. The Embarcadero	Easy	3.0	1.5
6. Fisherman's Wharf	Easy	3.5	2
7. Marina Green	Easy	3.75	2
8. Golden Gate Promenade	Easy	4.0	2
Pacific Coast			
9. Golden Gate Bridge and Baker Beach	Moderate	4.0	2.5
10. Ocean Beach	Easy	1.9	1
11. Lands End	Moderate	5.0	3
Other Distinctive Neighborhoods			
12. Pacific Heights and Japantown	Moderate	3.6	2
13. The Castro District and Noe Valley	Strenuous	4.1	2.5
14. Mission Murals	Easy	2.0	1

Trip Planner			
Walk	Difficulty	Distance (miles)	Time (hours)
Parklands			
15. Golden Gate Park	Easy	3.0	1.5
16. The Presidio	Moderate	3.1	1.5
17. Wolf Ridge Loop in the Marin Headlands	Strenuous	6.5	3.5
18. Rodeo Lagoon	Easy	1.5	1

Meet San Francisco
Fast Facts
General
County: San Francisco
Time zone: Pacific
Area code: 415

Size
Nation's fifth-largest metropolitan region
825,863 people within the city and county of San Francisco (2012 census estimate)
7.1 million people live in the nine-county metropolitan area
16.5 million visitors annually
About 47 square miles

Elevation
Sea level to 938 feet (Mount Davidson, with the Twin Peaks pulling a close second)

Climate
Average yearly precipitation: 23.64 inches
Average relative humidity, early morning: 85.8 percent
Average relative humidity, midday: 64 percent
Maximum average temperature: 63.9°F
Minimum average temperature: 51°F

Major Industries
Tourism, recreation, retail, transportation, publishing, technology, finance, construction, food, banking, biotechnology

Parks and Recreation
San Francisco is park-rich, with more than 1,000 city, county, and state parks, recreation centers, golf courses, swimming pools, public works of art, and stairways, plus the Golden Gate National Recreation Area, which encompasses more than 75,000 acres and about 60 miles of coastline.

Media
There's no shortage of broadcast entertainment available in the San Francisco Bay Area. What follows is just a small selection of stations that provide local coverage and/or local entertainment. Employ cable or satellite connections, and you've got the world at your fingertips.

Television Stations
KTVU (Fox; channel 2)
KRON (NBC; channel 4)
KPIX (CBS; channel 5)

KGO (ABC; channel 7)
KQED (PBS; channel 9)
KDTV (Univision; channel 14)

Radio Stations
KABL 960 AM—Big band
KCBS 740 AM—All news
KGO 810 AM—News, talk, and sports
KVTO 1400 AM—Asian
KIQI 1010 AM—Multicultural programming with a focus on the Hispanic community
KSOL 98.9 FM—Spanish
KUSF 90.3 FM—Alternative music
KCSM 91.1 FM—Jazz
KQED 88.5 FM—National Public Radio
KPOO 89.5 FM—Listener-sponsored public radio
KALW 91.7 FM—National Public Radio, BBC, CBC
KFOG 104.5 FM—Classic rock

Newspapers
San Francisco Bay Guardian (sfbg.com), *San Francisco Chronicle* (sfchronicle.com), *The San Francisco Examiner* (sfexaminer.com), *SF Weekly* (sfweekly.com), and many others, including papers in Chinese, Japanese, Korean, Spanish, German, and Russian, serve the various communities found in San Francisco.

Special Events
- January: Berlin and Beyond Film Festival, Dr. Martin Luther King Jr. Birthday Celebration
- February: Chinese New Year Parade and Celebration, San Francisco Tribal, Folk & Textile Art Show

- March: San Francisco Flower and Garden Show, CAAMFest (formerly the San Francisco International Asian American Film Festival)
- April: New Living Expo, Cherry Blossom Festival, San Francisco International Film Festival
- May: Carnaval in the Mission, Cinco de Mayo, San Francisco Youth Arts Festival, Bay to Breakers footrace
- June: Ethnic Dance Festival, Haight Ashbury Street Fair, Juneteenth Celebration, North Beach Festival, San Francisco Gay/Lesbian/Transgender Pride Celebration Parade, Union Street Spring Festival Arts & Crafts Fair
- July: Fillmore Jazz Festival, Jewish Film Festival, Fourth of July Waterfront Fireworks, Stern Grove Midsummer Music Festival
- August: American Craft Council Craft Fair, AfroSolo Arts Festival, Nihonmachi Street Fair, Outside Lands Music and Arts Festival
- September: Autumn Moon Festival, Comedy Celebration Day, Sea Music Festival, Folsom Street Fair, San Francisco Fringe Festival, San Francisco Shakespeare Festival
- October: The Grand National Livestock Exposition (locally known as the Grand National Rodeo), Horse Show, and Livestock Show; Halloween San Francisco; Hardly Strictly Bluegrass Festival; International Vintage Poster Fair; Italian Heritage Parade; LitQuake (San Francisco's Literary Festival); San Francisco Antiques Show; San Francisco Jazz Festival; Castro Street Fair

- November: Dia de los Muertos, American Indian Film Festival, Harvest Festival and Christmas Crafts Show, San Francisco International Automobile Show
- December: Festival of Lights and Lighted Boat Parade at Fisherman's Wharf, Christmas at Sea

Weather

San Francisco's temperate climate makes the city ideal for walking. With temperatures seldom dipping below 40°F and rarely rising above 70 (though there are occasional hot days), walking San Francisco is almost always cool and pleasant. Of course, you may be surprised by a heavy rainstorm in winter; if in doubt, carry a small umbrella in your jacket pocket, rucksack, or briefcase.

Weather-wise, spring and fall are the best times to visit the City by the Bay. December, January, and February are often rainy, and summer days, oddly enough, can chill you to the bone with wind and fog. Of course, most tourists come to San Francisco in the summer—another reason to visit in glorious October or radiant May—when the usual tourist spots are less crowded.

Because of topography, this city has several distinct microclimates. When Ocean Beach is drenched in fog, the Mission District can be sunny and bright. San Francisco's weather shifts moods within a few blocks. Walking the city means being prepared for a range of eventualities. Always carry that umbrella, and wear several layers. A heavy sweatshirt or light fleece jacket is the optimal outer layer and is easy to tie about your waist when the temperature rises.

Getting Around
Major Highways
- Interstates: I-80, I-280
- US highways: US 101
- State highways: CA 1, CA 35

By car: San Francisco is a challenging place to drive a car. Steep hills, narrow streets, constant traffic that compounds exponentially in morning and evening rush hours, and tremendous competition for on-street parking are compounded by bridge-crossing bottlenecks to the north at the Golden Gate Bridge and to the east at the Bay Bridge. If you can, stow your car and rely on public transportation to get around. Traffic is heaviest from 7 to 10 a.m. and from 4 to 7 p.m., but it is increasingly thick at all hours of the day.

Three major freeways offer access to and through San Francisco from the north, south, and east.

US 101 leads south from the North Bay (Marin and Sonoma Counties) across the Golden Gate Bridge and then through San Francisco on three city streets—Lombard Street, Van Ness Avenue, and South Van Ness Avenue. It resumes as a freeway several blocks south of Market Street and continues southward past San Francisco International Airport onto the San Francisco Peninsula and into the South Bay.

I-80 runs west from the East Bay across the Bay Bridge and travels through the city north of the South of Market area. It then flows into US 101, which heads north up Van Ness Avenue toward the Golden Gate Bridge and south down the San Francisco Peninsula.

I-280 heads north from the San Francisco Peninsula directly into the South of Market area. I-280 north may be less congested than US 101 north, and its main exit into downtown San Francisco is easier to negotiate.

Note: As of early 2014, construction on a new configuration of the Presidio Parkway, replacing Doyle Drive as the southern approach to the Golden Gate Bridge, was under way. The new highway, complete with seismic retrofitting and easier access to the waterfront, the Presidio, and Lombard Street, is slated for completion in 2016. Visit presidioparkway.org for the most up-to-date information.

Bridges

The eight major bridges in the San Francisco Bay Area require tolls. Obtaining a FasTrak electronic toll tag (bayareafastrak.org) is the most expedient way to navigate across those bridges; no need to carry toll money. Cash

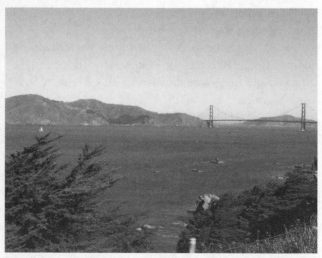

A walk on Lands End presents stellar views of the Golden Gate.

tolls are no longer collected at the Golden Gate Bridge; FasTrak is the best option, or the bridge will bill you based on your license plate/registration. Be sure to pay promptly, as penalties accumulate for unpaid tolls.

The most famous bridge is the Golden Gate Bridge (goldengatebridge.org), with the San Francisco–Oakland Bay Bridge (baybridgeinfo.org), boasting a new span that opened in 2013, pulling a close second. Other bridges include the Richmond–San Rafael Bridge, the Dumbarton Bridge, the Carquinez Bridge, and the San Mateo-Hayward Bridge.

Public Transportation

- Alameda–Contra Costa Transit District (AC Transit; actransit.org)
- Golden Gate Transit (goldengatetransit.org)
- Greyhound (greyhound.com)
- SamTrans (samtrans.com)
- San Francisco Municipal Transportation Agency (Muni; sfmta.com)
- To plan a trip using public transit, visit tripplanner .transit.511.org.

By bus: San Francisco has an excellent mass-transit system, the San Francisco Municipal Railway (Muni). Muni operates a fleet of electric- and diesel-powered buses that covers the entire city, the underground Muni Metro light-rail system, and the city's fabled cable cars and streetcars.

Muni schedules and maps are available from the San Francisco Visitors Bureau (www.sanfrancisco.travel) at Hallidie Plaza, or from selected merchants. Maps and schedules are also available online at sfmta.com. Many bus lines have wheelchair lifts; call Muni for details about accessibility.

Several regional bus lines link San Francisco with surrounding communities. Alameda–Contra Costa Transit District (AC Transit) buses run between San Francisco's Transbay Temporary Terminal and western Alameda and Contra Costa Counties in the East Bay. Golden Gate Transit buses cover Marin, Sonoma, San Francisco, and Contra Costa Counties. SamTrans serves San Mateo County with connections to Hayward, Palo Alto, and San Francisco's Transbay Temporary Terminal. Greyhound provides long-distance service to the city.

Note: The Transbay Temporary Terminal will be replaced by the new Transbay Transit Center (transbay center.org) at First and Mission, slated to open in 2017. In addition to serving as a hub for bus service, rail service provided by Caltrain, Amtrak, and a planned high-speed rail service linking San Francisco to Los Angeles will operate from the facility.

By cable car or streetcar: You're going to see them when you're walking, so you might as well hitch a ride on one. San Francisco's famous cable cars are a part of Muni, running on three separate lines: Powell-Hyde, Powell-Mason, and California Street. You may have to battle a tourist for a spot, but these historic cars are a great way to appreciate the city. For more information about the history of the cable car system, visit the Cable Car Barn and Museum at 1201 Mason (cablecarmuseum.org). Muni also operates several fleets of historic streetcars, which are powered by overhead electric cables. Contact Muni for ticket prices and schedules.

Airport Service

Most major airlines, both domestic and international, fly out of San Francisco International Airport (flysfo.com) or Oakland International Airport (flyoakland.com). Major carriers include Aero Mexico, Air Canada, Alaska Airlines, American Airlines, British Airways, Delta, Frontier Airlines, JetBlue, Southwest, United, and Virgin America.

By air: San Francisco International Airport (SFO) accommodates airlines from all over the world. It is located south of the city, outside San Bruno. Intriguing museum exhibits enliven passage through SFO—travelers have enjoyed everything from displays of African folk art to a history of the platform shoe. The airport's international terminal, completed in 2000, hosts not only exhibits but also a number of fine dining establishments.

Airport shuttles provide reliable, relatively inexpensive service to SFO from throughout the Bay Area. Some of the bigger shuttle companies—the Marin Airporter, for example—operate buses, which don't take you door to gate but are certainly cheaper than taxis.

Oakland International Airport, located across the Bay Bridge, is smaller and just as close to downtown San Francisco as SFO—about 30 minutes when traffic is not too heavy. Again, shuttles are a safe bet, although there is a designated bus—known as AirBART—that will take you to the nearest Bay Area Rapid Transit (BART) station for a quick underground jaunt into the city.

Rail Service

- Amtrak (amtrak.com)
- Caltrain (caltrain.com)
- Bay Area Rapid Transit (BART; bart.gov)

By train: Amtrak does not cross the bay into San Francisco, but you can find Amtrak passenger stations in Oakland, Emeryville, and Richmond. Amtrak buses transport passengers to and from San Francisco. Contact Amtrak for details (amtrak.com).

Bay Area Rapid Transit (BART) trains serve much of San Francisco, carrying commuters to and from East Bay cities like Oakland and Berkeley, and providing service from downtown to the Mission District. Caltrain provides commuter rail service between San Francisco and South Bay communities including Gilroy, with bus service continuing to Santa Cruz.

Ferry Service

- Blue & Gold Fleet (blueandgoldfleet.com)
- Golden Gate Ferry (goldengateferry.org)
- San Francisco Bay Ferry (sanfranciscobayferry.com)

By ferry: Although the Golden Gate and Bay Bridges have replaced ferries for many commuters, a number still take ferries into the city. Ferries departing from Pier 41 provide passage to Alameda/Oakland, Alcatraz, Angel Island, Sausalito, Tiburon, and Vallejo. Other ferries depart from the Ferry Building and provide service to Sausalito, Tiburon, Vallejo, Alameda, Oakland, and Larkspur.

Car and Bike Sharing

Ride sharing in San Francisco is not just about hitchhiking: You can also use Zipcars and cycles that are part of San Francisco's bike-share program. To use a Zipcar, call (415) 495-7478 or visit zipcar.com/sf. The San Francisco

Bicycle Coalition oversees a bike-share program; call (415) 431-BIKE or visit sfbike.org/?bikeshare.

Safety and Street Savvy

San Francisco is a friendly city, and San Franciscans take great delight in sharing their love for—and intimate knowledge of—the city with visitors. At the same time, San Francisco is not immune from the crime that plagues any large metropolitan area. But safety does not have to be your overriding concern when walking in San Francisco.

Safety mishaps in any large city, including San Francisco, are likely to involve petty theft or vandalism. The biggest tip is simple: Do not tempt thieves. Purses dangling on shoulder straps or slung over your arm, wallets peeking out of pockets, arms burdened with packages, valuables left on the car seat—these things attract the pickpocket, purse snatcher, or thief. If you look like you could easily be relieved of your possessions, you may be.

Do not carry a purse. Put your money in a money belt or tuck your wallet into a deep pocket of your pants or skirt, or in a fanny pack that rides over your hip or stomach. Lock your valuables in the trunk of your car before you park and leave for your walk. Protect your camera by wearing the strap across your chest, not just over your shoulder. Better yet, put your camera in a backpack.

You also will be safer if you remember the following:

- Be aware of your surroundings and the people near you.
- Avoid parks or other isolated places at night.
- Walk with others.
- Walk in well-lit and well-traveled areas.

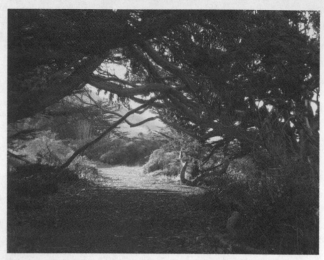

The sun filters through a bower of eucalyptus along the trail at Rodeo Lagoon in the Marin Headlands.

The walks in this book were selected with safety in mind. No walk will take you through a bad neighborhood or into an area of the city that is known to be dangerous. However, neighborhoods evolve. Let common sense be your guide. If you have concerns about a particular neighborhood or route, check with friends who live there or ask at the San Francisco Visitors Bureau. If you depart from a route, be aware that the character of a neighborhood can change within a few blocks.

In general, it is best to walk during the day. Daylight makes it easier to read maps and guidebooks, enjoy the sights, and see uneven surfaces on sidewalks and trails. We particularly recommend that you not take any walks in the Parklands or on the Pacific Coast after dark. In addition, on routes through less populated areas, such as in the

Parklands and along the Pacific Coast, it is recommended that you walk with a partner. If you do find yourself walking after dark, be sure to avoid alleyways, parks, and parking lots. When possible, choose well-lit thoroughfares.

A special note for water lovers: Swim only at beaches with lifeguards. Ocean swells and riptides, which can be extremely dangerous, are common along California's north coast and can catch the inexperienced off-guard. Information on tides and swells is published in local newspapers and available at tidesandcurrents.noaa.gov (search for San Francisco). Open-water swimming is available on the bay side at Aquatic Park, which is also the starting point for annual swimming events across the bay to Alcatraz Island.

The Story of San Francisco

San Francisco is blessed with a magnificent natural setting. With its great harbor, temperate climate, and proximity to prime agricultural lands and rich mineral deposits, it has—from its genesis—been destined to attract wealth, power, and creativity.

The Natives and the Colonists

The first humans known to have walked in San Francisco—the Coast Miwok and Ohlone—likely found the site of the present-day city relatively inhospitable. Faced with seemingly endless sand dunes, windswept cliffs, and steep hills, these hunter-gatherers found it easier to make a living farther inland, where game, fish, acorns from a variety of oaks, and edible wild plants were abundant, and the summertime fog was not quite so thick.

European explorers were relatively late in discovering the bay, resulting in a temporary respite for the native peoples they would later displace. For the first Spanish sailor to explore the California coast in 1542, and for the Spanish, English, and Russian captains who sailed along the rugged northern California shoreline for the next 200 years, the entrance to San Francisco Bay—later dubbed the Golden Gate—remained hidden. Why? Best bet: the fog.

It was not until 1769 that Spaniard Gaspar de Portola, exploring northward as part of missionary Junipero Serra's foray into Alta California, stumbled upon the great bay while traveling overland. And finally, in 1775, Juan Manuel de Ayala, commanding the *San Carlos*, became the first European to sail through the Golden Gate. Ayala's men thoroughly explored and mapped the bay, realizing that they had discovered a well-sheltered harbor of world-class proportions.

The first Spanish settlers arrived in 1776. In that year they established a military presence—a presidio—on the windy site of present-day Fort Point. They founded a Franciscan mission—Mission San Francisco de Asis (known as Mission Dolores)—3 miles to the southeast, in a valley sheltered from the wind and with plenty of water. They also founded a pueblo, which they named Yerba Buena ("good herb") after a creeping mint known for its healing properties. San Francisco's founding was celebrated with a Catholic mass on June 29, 1776, only five days before the ratification of the Declaration of Independence.

As old and as young as the American republic, San Francisco grew slowly at first. Not long a Spanish outpost, it became a part of Mexico following Mexican independence in 1821. On July 9, 1846, soon after war broke out between Mexico and the United States, a small American force took possession of Yerba Buena. San Francisco became American property—just in time for a gold rush that would transform what was a tiny community by the bay.

The Golden Transformation

With the discovery of gold at Sutter's Mill in the foothills of the Sierra Nevada in 1848, San Francisco morphed from sleepy village to rough-and-ready boomtown virtually overnight. Its grand harbor filled with ships, many of which were abandoned shortly after they arrived when their gold-fever-struck crews headed for the hills. The town's population shot from about 500 in 1847 to about 20,000 by the end of 1849. In an economy where gold was plentiful and merchandise of any sort—clothing, lumber, food—was in limited supply, San Francisco's entrepreneurs made instant fortunes. Levi Strauss blue jeans, for example, is an entrepreneurial brand with gold rush origins.

San Francisco's population in those boisterous days was made up mostly of single men, and many indulged in legendary drinking and gambling bouts. But, as with much of the frontier West, San Francisco rode a boom-and-bust economy. In 1855, with the gold of the Sierra harder and harder to exploit, the city suffered its first depression. To make matters worse, six major fires swept the city in its early years. But as the gold ran out, ranching, banking, and the construction trade diversified the region's economy. And in 1859 another mineral discovery, this time silver, in nearby Nevada's Comstock Lode, returned the city to boom times.

The Comstock Lode, centered in Virginia City, Nevada, not far from Lake Tahoe, brought vast wealth to San Francisco. Enterprising San Francisco businessmen invested profitably in the Virginia City mines, and the city's merchants outfitted the miners. Other forward-looking San Franciscans, including Leland Stanford, helped build the transcontinental railroad, linking the city with the East Coast. These tycoons built enormous mansions to celebrate their successes, and the city center soon featured magnificent hotels, business centers, and other emblems of a thriving economy. Drawn by the boom, tens of thousands of Chinese immigrants flocked to California to work on the railroad, many settling permanently in San Francisco.

After the Influx

The city suffered another economic downturn that lasted for most of the 1870s. But San Francisco's diversified economy recovered, and by the 1880s the city was vibrant. The harbor served a vast and fertile agricultural region, its shipping fleet delivering wheat and other goods to ports around the world. The city was a great whaling center for more than two decades, and whalers, cargo ships, ferries, yachts, and a fishing fleet kept the harbor busy.

To maximize ease of transport within San Francisco itself, a revolutionary cable car system was built to carry citizens and visitors up and down the city's steep hills. And in 1894, to celebrate its good fortune, the city put on a world's fair, the Midwinter Exposition. Held in Golden Gate Park, the fair hosted more than two million tourists and city residents.

Trial by Temblor and Fire

The city was transformed in 1906. On April 18, at 5:12 a.m., a powerful earthquake, estimated to have registered between 7.7 and 7.9 on the Richter scale, shook San

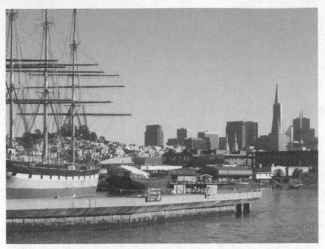

San Francisco's waterfront includes this view from the Municipal Pier in Aquatic Park.

Francisco and the surrounding region. The temblor, which lasted a minute, created a rupture almost 300 miles long along the northern California coast and brought down many of the city's wood, brick, and stone buildings.

Devastating in its own right, the earthquake initiated an even greater disaster: Several quake-caused fires coalesced to form a firestorm, which reached temperatures of nearly 2,000°F and consumed an estimated 28,000 buildings in 500 blocks. With most of the city's water mains broken, firefighters faced a hopeless task, and within three days about 250,000 citizens—out of a population of 400,000—lost their homes. Between the quake and the fire, an estimated 450 San Franciscans perished, though that number is debated and could be much higher. The elegant downtown, except for a handful of buildings, was razed.

In photographs taken immediately after the fire, San Francisco's cityscape resembles those of Dresden and Hiroshima after the firestorms of World War II. With 2,800 acres burned to the ground, rebuilding presented an enormous task. But with aid from around the world, the positive spirit of its citizens, and significant insurance settlements, the city built itself back up. A large percentage of the structures you see in today's San Francisco were constructed immediately following the disaster.

In 1915 San Francisco hosted another world's fair, this one known as the Panama-Pacific International Exposition. The grand exposition celebrated both the opening of the Panama Canal and San Francisco's resurrection. In what is now the Marina District, city engineers built a seawall and constructed the spectacular fairgrounds on sandy fill—setting the stage for more earthquake trouble in 1989.

Riding the Changing Tides

As elsewhere, the Great Depression of the 1930s brought hardship to San Francisco. At the same time, public building projects funded through the New Deal provided jobs and created new Bay Area landmarks. Prominent among these construction projects were two remarkable feats of engineering, the Golden Gate Bridge and the Bay Bridge.

With the outbreak of World War II, San Francisco's fortunes revived. Bay Area shipyards began producing ships of all kinds for the war effort, and military outposts on the bay prepared to defend the city from enemy attack. The shipyards, working around the clock, produced many hundreds of ships, especially the huge cargo vessels known as Liberty ships. Military installations dating back to the

Civil War line San Francisco Bay's shorelines, from Fort Point and the batteries on the bluffs overlooking the Golden Gate to Nike missile sites in the Marin Headlands. Luckily, the city's defenders have never had to fire a shot.

After World War II San Francisco indulged in some wild and controversial times. The 1950s and 1960s found the city—long known for its tolerance of the unconventional—a perfect testing ground for countercultural energies. The Beatniks brought a creative revolution to the North Beach neighborhood, and artists around the Bay Area continue to push the limits of literature, music, and the visual arts. Hippies brought the Summer of Love to the Haight-Ashbury, confirming San Francisco's place as a mecca for free spirits. And gay, lesbian, and transgender activists fought for equality in the Castro, where today same-sex couples walk hand in hand without fear of prejudice or judgment. The legacy of these movements is a city that remains vibrant, tolerant, and culturally fertile.

Boom, Then Bust, Then Boom Again

San Francisco has continued to suffer from occasional economic downturns, including one in the late 1980s. Adding insult to injury, another major earthquake struck in 1989, damaging area freeways and turning the fill upon which the Marina District was built to jello.

But the city hitched itself up again, and in the 1990s San Francisco experienced another boom. This time the treasures were virtual: technological marvels—software, hardware, innovations on the Internet—concocted by the digital alchemists of nearby Silicon Valley. As of this writing the technology boom remains a major economic force (along with biotechnology) in the region. The Bay Area's prospects for generating wealth seem limitless.

A commentator has called San Francisco "The New Rome." Certainly, the most recent influx of money and talent has given fresh energy to the city's cultural and civic institutions. City Hall and the city's opera house have undergone spectacular renovations; many of the city's museums have built or are building new homes; palm trees line the spruced-up Embarcadero; and a revitalized public library features state-of-the-art information technology. Already famous for its food, San Francisco has boasted more restaurants per capita than any other American city—by some counts the number of eateries tops 4,000.

San Francisco remains—with its stunning natural setting, richly textured urban fabric, and excellent mass transit system—a most congenial American city for walkers to explore.

HEART OF THE CITY

Walk 1: Downtown

🏢 👫 🛒 🍴

General location: In northeastern San Francisco, encompassing downtown and part of the South of Market district
Special attractions: Museums and theaters; shopping and restaurants; urban landscapes with varied architecture; gardens and parks; public monuments and pieces of art
Difficulty: Easy. The route is flat and entirely on sidewalks.
Distance: 3.3 miles
Estimated time: 2 hours
Services: Hotels, restaurants, restrooms, visitor information center
Restrictions: Not wheelchair accessible. Dogs must be leashed and their droppings picked up. This is a densely packed urban setting; sidewalks are often jammed with people.
For more Information: The San Francisco Travel Association, 900 Market St., Hallidie Plaza, San Francisco, CA 94102-2804; (415) 391-2000; sanfrancisco.travel
Getting started: This walk begins at the main entrance of the Grand Hyatt San Francisco Hotel, located at 345 Stockton St., 1 block north of Union Square. GPS: N37 47.362' / W122 24.413'

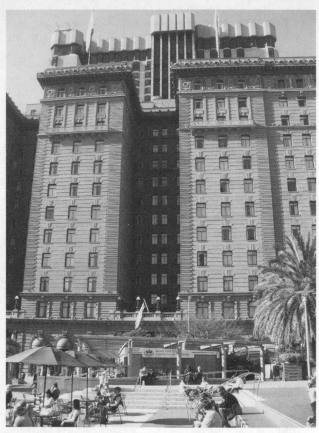

The swanky Westin St. Francis Hotel borders the west side of historic Union Square.

(1) From the intersection of Market, Third, Kearny, and Geary Streets, go 2 blocks north on Kearny. Go left on Sutter Street and continue for 2 blocks. Turn right onto Stockton Street, and then take an immediate right into the

entrance of the Sutter-Stockton Garage, one of the least expensive parking facilities close to Union Square.

(2) From the Golden Gate Bridge, continue south on US 101/Presidio Parkway, staying right onto Lombard Street. Drive about 1 mile on Lombard Street, then turn right on Van Ness Avenue, and go 14 blocks. Turn left on Bush Street and go 9.5 blocks. One and a half blocks past the intersection of Bush and Powell Streets, just beyond the bridge over the Stockton Street Tunnel, turn right into the entrance of the Sutter-Stockton Garage.

To reach the Grand Hyatt San Francisco Hotel from the Sutter-Stockton Garage, exit the garage onto Stockton Street, turn left, cross Sutter, and then cross Stockton to arrive at the hotel entrance.

Parking is also available at the Union Square Garage, which is beneath Union Square. Its entrance is on Geary Street. You will also find parking at the Fifth & Mission/Yerba Buena Gardens Garage at Fifth and Mission Streets, 1 block south of Market Street.

Public transportation: Numerous San Francisco Municipal Railway (Muni) bus lines and Muni Metro lines run past or near Union Square. All Bay Area Rapid Transit (BART) lines stop at Market and Powell Streets, 3 blocks south of Union Square. AC Transit and Golden Gate Transit buses stop at the Transbay Terminal.

Overview: Thriving without interruption since it was rebuilt after the 1906 fire, downtown San Francisco feels old-fashioned and up-to-the-minute at the same time. At its heart is Union Square, a dollop of open space amid the canyons of high-rise hotels and mercantiles. It may be compact, but the city's downtown encompasses enough enterprise, entertainment, and humanity to rival any downtown in the world.

This city's shoppers have not abandoned the city center for the seductions of suburban malls, and so the blocks around Union Square remain commercially vibrant. The retail mix includes art galleries, the city's most venerable hotels and department stores, and luxury specialty shops. Cartier, Armani, Gucci, Hermès of Paris, and the legendary Gump's are among them. You will also find a host of upscale mass retailers—Williams-Sonoma, Crate & Barrel, Banana Republic, Sur la Table, Gap—several of which got their start in the Bay Area.

This urban walk leads through downtown's retail mecca and skims the northern reaches of South of Market (SoMa), a dynamic neighborhood that has metamorphosed from industrial district to an outpost of the digital revolution. The area encompasses AT&T Park, home of the San Francisco Giants, as well as trendy nightclubs and restaurants, and the largest concentration of museums in the city. The San Francisco Museum of Modern Art (closed for construction/expansion until 2016) is a must-see destination on this walk, and just across Third Street from the museum, Yerba Buena Gardens offer multiple pleasures, from public art to sidewalk cafes to grassy knolls on which to recline after your long trek through crowded city streets.

The Walk

▶Start at the front door of the Grand Hyatt San Francisco Hotel at the corner of Stockton and Sutter Streets.

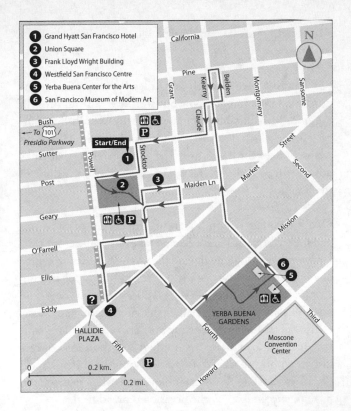

1. Grand Hyatt San Francisco Hotel
2. Union Square
3. Frank Lloyd Wright Building
4. Westfield San Francisco Centre
5. Yerba Buena Center for the Arts
6. San Francisco Museum of Modern Art

California

N

Pine

Bush

← To ⟨101⟩ /
Presidio Parkway

Start/End

Sutter

Post

Geary

O'Farrell

Ellis

Eddy

HALLIDIE
PLAZA

Powell

Stockton

Grant

Kearny

Claude

Belden

Montgomery

Sansome

Street

Market

Second

Maiden Ln

Mission

YERBA BUENA
GARDENS

Fourth

Third

Moscone
Convention
Center

Howard

Fifth

0   0.2 km.
0   0.2 mi.

▸Walk 1 block downhill on Stockton to Post Street, passing the circular fountain that San Francisco artist Ruth Asawa designed to "show what many hands working together can do." The scenes of San Francisco life depicted on this monument were modeled in bread dough by visitors to San Francisco and by more than one hundred children, and then cast in bronze.

▸Turn right onto Post and walk 1 block, passing Saks Fifth Avenue.

▸At Powell Street turn left and cross Post to arrive at the northwest corner of Union Square. The tall building in the middle of this block of Powell is the Westin St. Francis Hotel, a San Francisco landmark built in 1904 and restored after the 1906 fire. The cable car line that links downtown to Fisherman's Wharf passes the front door of the hotel.

▸Walk through Union Square to the corner of Stockton and Geary Streets. Union Square takes its name from pro-Union rallies held here during the Civil War. At the center of the square stands the Victory Monument, celebrating Commodore George Dewey's 1898 triumph over the Spanish fleet at Manila Bay. Street merchants and musicians station themselves at the corners of the square, and you may happen upon an outdoor art show or concert in this public space. Want to see some wildlife? Union Square harbors flocks of that ubiquitous urban denizen the pigeon, encouraged by the occasional bread feeder.

▸Cross Stockton and turn left, walking half a block uphill to Maiden Lane. To your left, at the edge of Union Square, is the kiosk for TIX Bay Area (tixbayarea.org), which sells half-price, day-of-performance tickets to theater, dance, and music events throughout the city. Full-price, advance sale tickets are also available here. San Francisco's theater district lies on the west side of Union Square, bounded by Powell, Geary, Sutter, and Taylor Streets.

THE HISTORIC F MARKET STREETCAR LINE

Cable cars are a signature San Francisco attraction. But walking through downtown, you will also encounter the cable cars' lesser-known cousins: the bright-colored electric cars of the F Market & Wharves Streetcar Line.

Tracing its origins to 1860, horse cars, steam engines, cable cars, and streetcars have run on the Market Street tracks. Not just a piece of nostalgia, the F Market Line offers a delightful aboveground alternative to the subterranean Muni Metro lines.

A virtual inventory of disappearing electric streetcar systems worldwide, the F Market railway runs vintage cars from Australia, Italy, and Japan. Some of its historic streetcars sport the eye-catching color schemes of American electric railways no longer in existence, like the Pacific Electric Red Car. Market Street Railway (streetcar.org), a volunteer group founded in 1976, actively acquires and donates vintage streetcars to the San Francisco Municipal Railway (Muni). The volunteers also pitch in to help Muni restore and maintain its fleet of historic cars. Unlike San Francisco's famous cable cars, the F Market railway is powered by an overhead electrical cable, as are some city buses and other streetcar lines.

The F Market Line runs every day along Market Street between the Transbay Temporary Terminal and Castro Street. For information about routes and stops on the F Market line and other electric lines in the city, contact Muni.

▸Turn right into Maiden Lane and walk 1 block. The "maidens" of San Francisco's bawdy post–gold rush nightlife once dominated this dark alley, which is now a narrow, pedestrian-only street lined with small restaurants and elegant shops. Cafe tables spill out into the street, and shoppers can reenergize with a salad, a chunk of San Francisco sourdough bread, and a glass of wine.

The striking building at 140 Maiden Ln. was remodeled in 1949 by master architect Frank Lloyd Wright. Faithfully restored in every detail in 1998, this architectural jewel—with its spiraling ramp—recalls on a much more intimate scale Wright's Guggenheim Museum of 1943. This landmark, now housing an Asian art gallery, is definitely worth a visit.

▸Turn right onto Grant Avenue and continue for half a block to Geary, passing several specialty stores.

▸Turn right onto Geary and walk west, back toward Union Square. Britex Fabrics, midway along the block, boasts an inventory of textiles so large that it requires four floors to house it all.

▸At the corner of Geary and Stockton Streets, turn left and cross to the opposite side of Geary (to the entrance of Neiman Marcus) and then turn right and cross Stockton. The flower stands gracing these corners are a San Francisco tradition, adding sweetness and color to this crowded commercial intersection for more than 40 years.

▸Turn left onto Stockton and walk downhill, passing the entrance to Macy's San Francisco on your right and Macy's Men's Store on your left.

▸Turn right onto O'Farrell Street and walk 1 block to Powell.

▸Cross Powell, turn left, and walk downhill on Powell for 2 blocks to Market Street. The turntable for the cable car that negotiates the steep hills between downtown and Fisherman's Wharf is at the intersection of Market and Powell. This area is often congested with people lining up to buy cable car tickets or to watch the cable cars make the turn. San Francisco Travel's visitor center is also near this corner, below street level and outside the Powell Street BART / Muni Metro station. Look for the signs for BART, take the escalator down to the lower level of Hallidie Plaza, and cross the brick courtyard to the visitor center. Pick up an armload of brochures and get your questions answered, then ride the escalator back up to the corner of Powell and Market. Look up and down Market Street to catch glimpses of the historic F Market & Wharves Streetcar Line.

▸Cross Market Street. A few hundred feet to your right, at the corner of Fifth and Market Streets, is the entrance to Westfield San Francisco Centre, a vertical shopping mall with ninety upscale retail stores. It is noted for the escalator that spirals up through its central atrium.

▸Turn left onto Market and walk 1 block to Fourth Street.

YERBA BUENA GARDENS

The 10 acres of Yerba Buena Gardens count among San Francisco's most appealing open spaces. Here, in midst of the noisy South of Market area, you'll find sanctuary from the urban hustle and bustle and enjoy a rich array of cultural offerings.

Set atop a part of the giant Moscone Convention Center and just across the street from the San Francisco Museum of Modern Art, Yerba Buena Gardens encompass Yerba Buena Center for the Arts, including art galleries and forums for the performing arts and theater. Other attractions include an outdoor stage, a collection of public sculptures, and plenty of handsomely landscaped green space encircled by a paved esplanade.

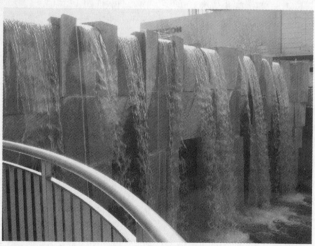

The waterfall memorial dedicated to the memory of Dr. Martin Luther King, Jr. at Yerba Buena Gardens.

Yerba Buena Gardens have expanded since they first opened in 1993. A special feature is Reiko Goto's butterfly garden—on the northeastern edge of the esplanade—made up of plantings congenial to several species of butterflies native to the Bay Area. Another unique garden, on the upper terrace of the esplanade, honors San Francisco's thirteen sister cities around the globe and features flowering plants from each. The centerpiece of the gardens—a stone and glass memorial to Martin Luther King Jr.—offers a powerful message of peace and hope.

Learn more about Yerba Buena Gardens, including upcoming events, at yerbabuenagardens.com.

▶Cross Fourth, turn right, and walk along Fourth for 1 block to Mission Street.

▶Cross Mission, turn left, and walk one-half block along Mission. The vast Metreon mall, with its shops and theaters, dominates this block.

▶Turn right into Yerba Buena Gardens; you've walked about 1.5 miles at this point. Walk to the waterfall memorial to Dr. Martin Luther King Jr. at the center of the gardens. In the shade of the grotto behind the waterfall, you can pause to read King's words, translated into the many languages of San Francisco's residents.

▶Take the ramp to the right of the waterfall to the upper level, which overlooks the garden and offers cafe seating on its terrace. Beyond and across Third Street, you will see the distinctive striped tower of the San Francisco Museum of

Modern Art. St. Patrick Church is across Mission, in the shadow of the towering San Francisco Marriot Marquis.

▶Walk down the ramp leading from the end of the balcony closest to Third Street.

▶Turn right and walk past the large glass sculpture of a boat hull, called *Seasons of the Sea Adrift*. Exit the gardens onto Third.

▶Cross with the light to the entrance of the San Francisco Museum of Modern Art. The museum, relocated in 1995 from the Civic Center area to this site in South of Market, has been instrumental in extending the reach of San Francisco's downtown into this light industrial and warehouse district. Its permanent collection focuses on modern and contemporary art. The museum building, inspired by the Modernist tradition, was designed by Swiss architect Mario Botta. Particularly impressive are the spacious and skylit galleries on the top floor, and the bridge and circular stairway leading down from these galleries. The museum also has a fine gift shop with an emphasis on art books. Expansion of the museum was under way in 2014, when this book was revised. Expected to reopen in 2016, the renovation will double the museum's exhibit space. During the construction, the museum gift shop is on Yerba Buena Lane, across from the gift shop for the Contemporary Jewish Museum.

▶Turn left and walk 1.5 blocks on Third toward Market.

▶Cross Market. You are now at the intersection of Kearny, Geary, and Market Streets.

▶Walk north on Kearny, away from Market Street, for 3 blocks.

▶Turn right onto Bush Street and then, after a short quarter block, turn left into Belden Place, a gathering spot within San Francisco's European Quarter. Tucked into this tiny alley is a collection of smart French and Italian restaurants in a setting reminiscent of Montmartre in Paris. If the weather is good, the alley is crowded with people partaking of the quintessential Parisian pastime of lingering at an outdoor table as the afternoon shadows grow long.

▶Exit Belden Place onto Pine Street and turn left, walking up to Kearny Street. Cross Kearny and go left, following Kearny 1 block to Bush Street.

▶Cross Bush Street and turn right, following Bush for a quarter block. Turn left into Claude Lane, another locus of the European Quarter and home to a small French restaurant.

▶Walk through Claude Lane to its opening onto Sutter Street.

▶Turn right onto Sutter and walk 2 blocks to Stockton, passing a number of art galleries and well-known specialty retailers, including the flagship store of Banana Republic. Many of the galleries are not on ground level; watch for their names on the brass nameplates at building entrances.

▶Cross Stockton, turn left, and cross Sutter to return to the Grand Hyatt San Francisco Hotel and the end of this walk.

Walk 2: Chinatown

🏢 👫 🛒 ✕

General location: In northeastern San Francisco, between the downtown shopping district and North Beach

Special attractions: Chinese cultural sites; historic architecture; shopping and restaurants; parks and public art

Difficulty: Easy. Keep in mind that the sidewalks are often extremely crowded. You will also climb a few short hills.

Distance: 1.8 miles

Estimated time: 1 hour

Services: Restaurants, restrooms

Restrictions: Not wheelchair accessible. Dogs must be leashed and their droppings picked up.

For more information: The San Francisco Travel Association, 900 Market St., Hallidie Plaza, San Francisco, CA 94102-2804; (415) 391-2000; sanfrancisco.travel. The Chinese Culture Center of San Francisco, 750 Kearny St., Third Floor, San Francisco, CA 94108; (415) 986-1822; c-c-c.org. The Chinese Historical Society of America, 965 Clay St., San Francisco, CA 94108; (415) 391-1188; chsa.org.

Getting started: This walk begins at the gate to Chinatown at the junction of Bush Street and Grant Avenue. GPS: N37 47.438' / W122 24.342'

(1) From the intersection of Market, Third, Kearny, and Geary Streets, travel north 2 blocks on Kearny. Go left onto Sutter Street, and continue for 2 blocks. Turn right onto Stockton Street, and then take an immediate right into the entrance of the Sutter-Stockton Garage, one of the least expensive parking facilities close to Union Square.

(2) From the Golden Gate Bridge, continue south on US 101/Presidio Parkway, staying right onto Lombard Street. Drive about 1 mile east on Lombard Street, then turn right onto Van Ness Avenue, and go 14 blocks. Turn left onto Bush Street and go 9.5 blocks. One and a half blocks past the intersection of Bush and Powell Streets, just beyond the bridge over the Stockton Street Tunnel, turn right into the entrance of the Sutter-Stockton Garage.

To reach the Chinatown Gate from the Sutter-Stockton Garage, exit the garage onto Sutter Street, turn left, and walk a partial block downhill to Grant. Turn left onto Grant, and walk 1 block uphill to the corner of Bush and Grant.

Parking is also available at the Union Square Garage beneath Union Square and at the Portsmouth Square Garage at Kearny and Clay Streets in Chinatown.

Public transportation: A number of San Francisco Municipal Railway (Muni) bus lines stop near the beginning of this walk. All Muni Metro and Bay Area Rapid Transit (BART) lines stop at Market and Powell Streets, 6 blocks from the Chinatown Gate. AC Transit and Golden Gate Transit bus lines stop at the Transbay Terminal at Mission and First Streets.

Overview: This stimulating walk takes you through one of San Francisco's most famous ethnic neighborhoods. Chinatown—situated between downtown San Francisco and the bohemian enclave of North Beach—is second only to Fisherman's Wharf as a destination for tourists visiting the City by the Bay.

This legendary community, where Chinese Americans maintain a clear cultural identity and many of the traditions of their homeland, is crowded and vibrant and endlessly intriguing. Here, along Grant Avenue and Stockton Street and in the narrow alleys of the neighborhood, you will find curio shops and restaurants aimed at tourists alongside the workaday establishments frequented by those who call Chinatown home.

Approximately 200,000 Chinese Americans live in San Francisco, and many live in Chinatown. The neighborhood is overcrowded, as you'll experience firsthand on this walk; as a result, immigrants from Vietnam and Hong Kong have settled in the Russian Hill, North Beach, Richmond, and Sunset districts. Still, Chinatown remains the epicenter for Chinese culture in the Bay Area.

This walk takes you beyond Chinatown's usual tourist byways. Within these few blocks, you will pass teahouses and temples, fish and fowl markets, merchants peddling fresh vegetables and dried herbs, florists and fortune-cookie manufacturers, benevolent associations and banking houses. Give yourself plenty of time to take in the sights, sounds, smells, and tastes of Chinatown.

The Walk

▶Start at the Chinatown Gate—complete with sculpted dragons—at the junction of Bush Street and Grant Avenue. The gate is just across Bush from San Francisco's tiny French Quarter and only a few blocks from downtown's Union Square.

▶Pass through the Chinatown Gate and head up Grant, the district's primary tourist thoroughfare. In this first block you will pass many curio shops and art galleries.

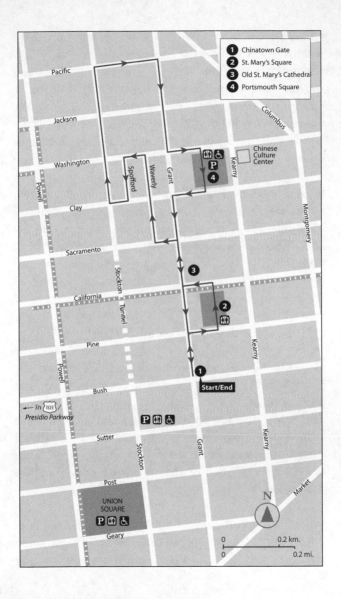

1. Chinatown Gate
2. St. Mary's Square
3. Old St. Mary's Cathedral
4. Portsmouth Square

Pacific

Jackson

Columbus

Washington

Chinese
Culture
Center

Spofford

Waverly

Grant

Kearny

4

Clay

Montgomery

Sacramento

Stockton

3

California

Tunnel

2

Pine

Powell

Bush

1
Start/End

To 101 /
Presidio Parkway

Sutter

Stockton

Grant

Kearny

Market

Post

UNION
SQUARE

Geary

N

0   0.2 km.

0   0.2 mi.

▶Walk 1 block to Pine Street. Cross Pine and turn right, walking down Pine to the entrance of St. Mary's Square midblock. Turn left into this small, quiet park, where you will find a public restroom, benches, and lawns. The monument that dominates the park, created by sculptor Benny Bufano, honors Dr. Sun Yat-sen, the reformer who led the 1911 revolution against the Manchu dynasty and established a modern republic in China.

▶Pass through St. Mary's Square and exit onto California Street. Take a left and walk up the hill to the corner of California and Grant. The striking church on California Street opposite St. Mary's Square is the old St. Mary's Cathedral. The brick walls and stone foundation of this landmark survived the 1906 earthquake and fire, and the remainder of the church was rebuilt. St. Mary's is one of several Christian churches in Chinatown, and is thought to be the oldest church in the neighborhood.

▶Cross California and continue down Grant, walking on the right side of the street. At the corner of Grant and Sacramento Street, look diagonally across the intersection to the large building on the corner. Colorful pagoda-like architecture, complete with upturned eaves, is perched atop the otherwise Western-style home of the Gold Mountain Monastery, run by the Dharma Realm Buddhist Association.

▶Cross Sacramento, then head up Sacramento for one-third block to Waverly Place. At the corner of Sacramento and Waverly (15 Waverly Place), you will see the Arts and

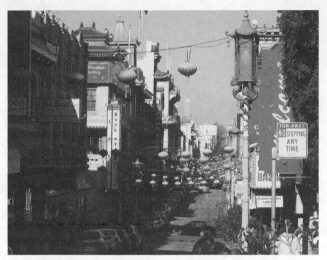

Festive colors and lanterns enliven a walk down Chinatown's Grant Avenue.

Crafts–style brick First Chinese Baptist Church, built in 1908 by architect G. E. Burlingame.

▶Take a right into Waverly Place, one of Chinatown's wonderful alleys and, since 1906, home to many of Chinatown's district and family associations. The people of Chinatown organized associations to aid fellow immigrants with everything from housing to burial costs. Family associations are organized around kinship, and the district associations benefit those who come from the same village or speak the same dialect. Associations remain a vital part of the Chinatown community.

In the first block of Waverly you will see several association headquarters. Note the Chinese-style decorative elements added to the top floors of these otherwise unassuming buildings.

▶Cross Clay Street and continue on Waverly. In the second block of Waverly, at 125 Waverly Place, on the left, is the Tin How Temple, a brightly decorated Taoist house of worship. This temple, with its intricately carved and gilded shrines, honors Tien Hau, the Taoist goddess of heaven and the sea, as well as other gods and legendary figures. Born with a "heart full of compassion and good virtue," Tien Hau was "destined to be the savior of the mortals." The first Tin How Temple in San Francisco was built in 1852, making this the oldest Chinese temple in the United States.

▶Depart Waverly at Washington Street, turning left to ascend a partial block to Spofford Alley.

▶Turn left into Spofford, also known as New Spanish Alley. As you walk down the narrow lane, listen for the gentle sound of mah-jongg tiles sliding across gaming tables from behind colorful closed doors.

Legend has it that Dr. Sun Yat-sen, first president of the Republic of China, lived in Spofford Alley when he came to San Francisco early in the twentieth century. He was the guest of the Chee Kung Tong, also known as the Chinese Freemasons. Note the sign for this association at 36 Spofford Alley.

▶At the end of Spofford Alley, turn right onto Clay Street and walk uphill one-third block to Stockton Street. At the corner of Stockton and Clay, look off to your left. At 843

Stockton, you will see the bright-colored headquarters of the powerful Chinese Consolidated Benevolent Association. Originally known as the Six Companies, the benevolent association looks after the political, legal, and cultural interests of the entire community. To the left of the Six Companies headquarters is Chinese Central High School, one of several private schools in Chinatown devoted to instructing students in Chinese language and culture.

▸Cross Stockton and turn right to walk on the uphill side of Stockton for 3 blocks to Pacific Avenue. Unlike Grant Avenue, Stockton was never intended to attract tourists. Instead, it serves as the main shopping street for Chinatown's residents. The street is lined with grocery stores, pastry shops, fishmongers, and poultry and meat markets, as well as herbal shops and acupuncturists.

Like Grant, Stockton is packed with humanity: Be patient and practice your urban-density dance, twisting and turning, always looking ahead for an opening, taking in the sometimes familiar, and more often completely unfamiliar, foodstuffs for sale. The dried products are provocative, but watching a Chinese matron walking down the street with two frogs dangling from a hand is something entirely different. Venture into shops, stop for a moment at street corners to survey the bustling scene, and admire the skill and good humor with which the local residents navigate their neighborhood.

▸Take a right onto Pacific and descend 1 block to Grant. Pass a Chinese-style housing project on the right; built in the 1950s, these apartments are painted red, green, and yellow, signifying happiness, health, and wealth in Chinese tradition.

▶Take a right onto Grant and walk 2 blocks to Washington Street.

▶Cross Washington and then turn left to walk down Washington. At midblock turn right into Portsmouth Square (1.3 miles). This historic park, a gathering place for the community, was originally the plaza for Yerba Buena (which translates as "good herb"), the Spanish pueblo that predated San Francisco. In 1846 Captain John B. Montgomery claimed Yerba Buena for the United States and named the plaza for his ship, USS *Portsmouth*. The Chinese Culture Center is located across Kearny Street; cross Kearny on the brick pedestrian bridge and take a few minutes to visit the cultural center's art exhibits and bookstore. A city-owned parking garage is on the lower level of Portsmouth Square.

▶Rest on Portsmouth Square's benches, if you can find space. On weekends the square may be packed with locals playing card games and chess. If the timing is right, you can catch a Chinese opera or musical performance. When you are ready to move on, walk through the park onto Clay Street, turn right, and head up the hill half a block to Grant.

▶Turn left onto Grant and walk 4 blocks to the Chinatown Gate and the end of this walk.

Walk 3: North Beach and Coit Tower

🏢 🛒 🍴 📷

General location: In northeastern San Francisco, adjoining the Embarcadero, Chinatown, and Russian Hill

Special attractions: Restaurants and coffeehouses; urban landscapes with varied architecture; bay and city views; literary landmarks; public art; parks

Difficulty: Strenuous, with several steep hills and flights of stairs

Distance: 2.3 miles

Estimated time: 1.5 hours

Services: Restaurants, restrooms

Restrictions: Not wheelchair accessible. Dogs must be leashed and their droppings picked up.

For more information: The San Francisco Travel Association, 900 Market St., Hallidie Plaza, San Francisco, CA 94102-2804; (415) 391-2000; sanfrancisco.travel

Getting started: This walk begins in Washington Square, at the corner of Union and Stockton Streets. GPS: N37 48.078' / W122 24.568'

(1) From the intersection of Market, Third, Kearny, and Geary Streets, go north 9.5 blocks on Kearny to Columbus Avenue. Turn left onto Columbus and go 4.5 blocks to Union Street. Turn right onto Union and go 1 block to the corner of Union and Stockton Streets.

(2) From the Golden Gate Bridge, continue south on US 101 / Presidio Parkway, staying right onto Lombard Street. Drive about 1 mile on Lombard Street to Van Ness

Avenue. Stay in the far left lane on Lombard, cross Van Ness, and continue on Lombard for 1 block to Polk Street. Turn right onto Polk and go 3 blocks. Turn left onto Union Street and go 8 blocks to the corner of Union and Stockton Streets.

On-street parking in this neighborhood is both scarce and time restricted. The many small lots and garages are expensive; one of the more reasonable is the Vallejo Street Garage at 766 Vallejo. Parking is also available in Chinatown at the Portsmouth Square Garage, on Kearny between Washington and Clay Streets. Using public transportation to get to Washington Square is highly recommended.

Public transportation: Several San Francisco Municipal Railway (Muni) buses stop on Washington Square near the starting point of this walk. Contact Muni for information about schedules, fares, and accessibility (sfmta.com, trip planner.transit.511.org).

Overview: This challenging walk, with its steep climbs and staircases, is one of San Francisco's most appealing. It starts out in peaceful Washington Square, in aromatic and trendy North Beach, where you can stoke the furnace before you climb and replenish after you descend. The first stop is the top of Telegraph Hill at Coit Tower, where the views are panoramic. Drop down a famous San Francisco stairway through luxuriant gardens, take a block-long breather, and then climb back up Telegraph Hill on another of those signature stairways.

The route then leads through the charming residential neighborhood on the lower slopes of Telegraph Hill and into the heart of North Beach, with its coffeehouses, boutiques, galleries, and vivid street life. The urban density in North Beach can rival that of neighboring Chinatown, but this is a neighborhood where European immigrants of many nationalities settled. North Beach was, for many years, an Italian enclave, and though it is now more ethnically diverse, the blocks surrounding Columbus Avenue retain a Mediterranean quality that is underscored by the neighborhood's numerous espresso bars, caffès, delis, and coffee roasters.

Like several other walks in this guide, this route showcases that particular San Francisco admixture of disparate cultures happily coexisting, of city life at its most exhilarating, and natural beauty at its most breathtaking.

The Walk

►Start in Washington Square, at the corner of Union and Stockton Streets. The square is a pleasant patch of green space at the foot of Telegraph Hill, open and quiet, perfect for lounging, family picnics, or reading a good book. Art exhibits and the occasional musical performance enliven the square.

►Leave Washington Square and cross Stockton Street, then take a left on Stockton. Saints Peter and Paul Church, one of San Francisco's most beautiful places of worship, dominates the Filbert Street side of the square. Begun in 1922 and completed in 1939, the Gothic Revival church is a spiritual touchstone in the North Beach community.

►Walk 3 blocks on Stockton, crossing Filbert and Greenwich Streets. Pass the North Beach Athletic Club and North Beach post office, plus several restaurants, coffeehouses, groceries, and bakeries. Liguria Bakery, at the

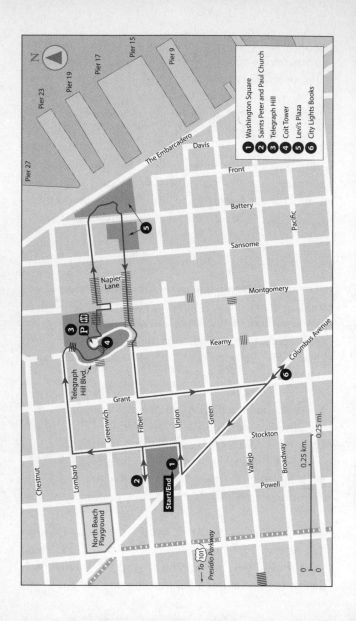

N

Pier 23
Pier 19
Pier 17
Pier 15
Pier 9
Pier 27

The Embarcadero
Davis
Front
Battery
Sansome
Pacific
Montgomery
Kearny
Columbus Avenue
Stockton
Vallejo
Broadway
Powell

Napier Lane

Telegraph Hill Blvd.
Grant
Greenwich
Filbert
Union
Green

Chestnut
Lombard

North Beach Playground

To 101
Presidio Parkway

Start/End

0.25 mi.
0.25 km.

1 Washington Square
2 Saints Peter and Paul Church
3 Telegraph Hill
4 Coit Tower
5 Levi's Plaza
6 City Lights Books

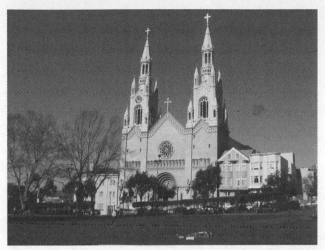

Saints Peter and Paul Church dominates the north side of
Washington Square.

corner of Stockton and Filbert, is famous for its focaccia,
and a line of customers sometimes snakes out the door.
Peer into the charming courtyard of the handsome building at 1736 Stockton, originally designed by renowned
Bay Area architect Bernard Maybeck.

▶At Lombard, the third cross street, turn right. Signs
direct you up Lombard toward Coit Tower. Climb 2 steep
blocks. Like most of the residential streets on Telegraph
Hill, Lombard is home to a pleasing mix of new and old
single-family dwellings, condominiums, and apartment
houses.

▶Just beyond Kearny Street, near the start of Telegraph
Hill Boulevard, Lombard stops abruptly at the edge of a
cliff. From this overlook, views extend out over the Bay

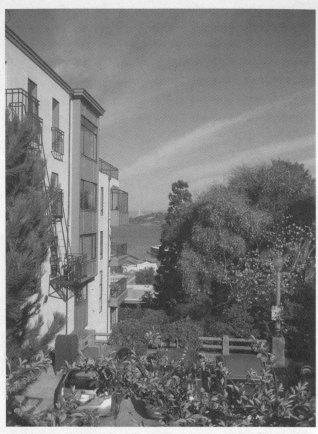
Looking north from the Filbert Street stairs on Telegraph Hill, you can see to the bay.

Bridge and the waterfront piers. On a clear day you can see Oakland and Berkeley across the bay.

▸Stairs ascend into a grove of cypress to the right. Take the stairs up onto a wide paved path that winds upward to the backside of Coit Tower. Leave the path after about 100 yards, taking a second set of stairs that breaks left. The stairs climb to the parking lot at the front of Coit Tower (0.7 mile).

►Circle the plaza surrounding the tower and take in the spectacular views, some of the finest in San Francisco. People from all over the world are drawn to Coit Tower, and on most days you can hear a veritable United Nations of languages spoken here.

►Enter the tower's front door to view the splendid murals created by twenty-five California artists during the 1930s. In the gift shop you may purchase tickets to tour the top of the tower, where you can enjoy 360-degree views of the City by the Bay.

►Upon leaving the tower, turn right and cross Telegraph Hill Boulevard. At the street sign for Greenwich Street, you will see the beginning of the Greenwich Street stairs. Descend the brick steps, which drop through towering trees and past beautifully tended gardens.

►The first "landing" of the stair-step descent is at Montgomery Street. The landmark restaurant Julius' Castle is on the left. Closed for several years and damaged by fire in 2013, the castle may be restored and reopened in the future. Pause and enjoy the extraordinary views from the overlook fronting the castle. Unless the fog is in, you'll see the marina at PIER 39, studded with sailboats, the easternmost half of Alcatraz Island, Treasure Island, and the

NORTH BEACH: A LITERARY PLACE

City Lights Books is not the only literary landmark in North Beach, and Lawrence Ferlinghetti is not the neighborhood's only poet, though he is one of San Francisco's poet laureates. But City Lights and Ferlinghetti embody North Beach literary traditions that stretch back to the 1950s and beyond.

In the district's coffeehouses and saloons, poets and writers including Ferlinghetti, Allen Ginsberg, Gary Snyder, Lew Welch, and Jack Kerouac started a revolution in American letters. On one fabled night in October 1955, Ginsberg read "Howl," a poem definitive of both the artist and the movement, to an ecstatic audience at Six Gallery, and San Francisco's poetry renaissance was on. Beat poets and their followers, dressed in hipster black, celebrated a new freedom of language and lifestyle in North Beach cafes and coffeehouses.

Some of the legendary Beat hangouts—Vesuvio Cafe, Tosca Cafe, Caffe Trieste, and the U.S. Restaurant—still operate today. Some, like the U.S. Restaurant, have been gentrified, their shabby charm stripped away in favor of a sleek 1990s look, but some still, in atmosphere and attitude, hark back to that wilder time.

Poetry readings and poetry slams are still part of the North Beach literary scene. Alleyways and side streets have been named in honor of the city's best-loved poets—Ferlinghetti, Kenneth Rexroth, Robert Duncan, Jack Spicer, Welch—most of whom spent time in North Beach. "Pulse after pulse came out of North Beach from the fifties forward," wrote Gary Snyder in a famous essay, "that touched the lives of people around the world."

Bay Bridge. Listen for the raucous chatter of the wild parrots of Telegraph Hill.

▶Turn right and walk alongside the overlook wall (on the bay side of the Montgomery Street loop) for thirty paces or so. In front of one of the residences, a sign marks the beginning of the 300 block of Greenwich Street. At the sign take a sharp left, and walk under a small overpass that belongs to the apartment house beside you. The Greenwich stairs continue down the hill, passing among modest bungalows, apartment buildings, and other private residences.

A series of lovely gardens spills alongside the staircase, lush with impatiens and roses, stalks of wild fennel, and expanses of nasturtium. Little rest stops with benches invite climbers to sit and rest a while. Keep an eye out for the Telegraph Hill parrots, with their brilliant red heads and green bodies. You'll likely see them perched in the trees or on telephone lines, and you will almost certainly hear their harsh voices.

▶Reach the bottom of the stairs at about 1.25 miles. Follow Greenwich Street to its intersection with Sansome Street. Cross Sansome and continue 1 block farther on Greenwich to Battery Street.

▶Take a right onto Battery Street. Pass Il Fornaio, an Italian restaurant and bakery on the right, a delightful place to refuel. Levi's Plaza, a small urban oasis, is beyond Il Fornaio, flanking Battery on both sides. Take a breather in the plaza, savoring the rush of running water in the fountains, the public sculptures, and beautifully groomed lawns. The corporate headquarters of Levi Strauss & Co., the well-known jeans-manufacturing company founded in the gold rush era, are housed in the handsome brick buildings that bound the plaza; the lobby of the glass-fronted main building of Levi Strauss & Co. features a display that recounts the company's colorful history.

▶Exit Levi's Plaza to the left of the largest fountain, onto Sansome Street. Cross Sansome and head for the exposed cliff straight ahead, where you will find the beginning of the Filbert Street steps.

▶Climb back up Telegraph Hill via the Filbert Street stairs. The steps lead through another luxuriant garden, this one named for Grace Marchant, its founder and guardian spirit. Cross quaint Napier Lane, one of the last boardwalk streets remaining in the city.

▶When you arrive at Montgomery Street, look left to the Art Deco apartment building at 1360 Montgomery. This elegant building was the setting for the 1947 film *Dark Passage*, starring Humphrey Bogart and Lauren Bacall.

▶Cross Montgomery to the continuation of the Filbert Street steps. Another set of steps amid lush landscaping leads up the hill toward Coit Tower, passing a mass of bougainvillea with fluorescent purple blooms, and then a sumptuous rose garden.

▸The stairs deposit you on Telegraph Hill Boulevard. Veer left and descend alongside the roadway to where Filbert meets Telegraph Hill Boulevard. Stay on the sidewalk and descend Filbert 1 block to Grant Avenue. Stairs down the middle of the sidewalk ease the steep descent.

▸At Grant take a left and walk 3.5 blocks through the vibrant, almost always crowded shopping district known locally as Upper Grant. You will pass small neighborhood groceries, pizza joints, coffeehouses, restaurants, bookstores, music emporiums, shops selling vintage and designer clothing, nightclubs, and the occasional purveyor of North Beach memorabilia. The Beat-era landmark Caffe Trieste—at Grant and Vallejo—offers one of the most powerful cappuccinos in the city.

▸When you reach the corner of Grant and Columbus Avenues, continue downhill on Columbus for a partial block and cross Broadway. Turn right and cross Columbus. Turn left and make your way to City Lights, the literary landmark, at 261 Columbus. City Lights was the epicenter of the Beat explosion in the 1950s. Founded by poet Lawrence Ferlinghetti, this world-class bookstore and publishing house remains a destination for every book lover who visits the city. Books line the shelves for three floors, and readers can browse for hours, as the store is open until midnight.

▶Once you have sated your bookish appetites, exit City Lights. Cross back to the corner of Broadway and Columbus, then proceed up Columbus toward Washington Square. These long, densely packed blocks are the very core of North Beach. Restaurants, Italian delis, curio shops, a seemingly endless string of atmospheric coffeehouses, and hundreds of fellow pedestrians enliven every step. Savor the sounds and smells of this bohemian pleasure ground. North Beach never fails to stimulate. Check out the plaque on the Condor Club at 560 Broadway, where the legendary stripper Carol Doda brought "topless and bottomless entertainment" to the city.

▶At the corner of Columbus and Union, cross both Columbus and Union to Washington Square. Walk down Union to the corner of Stockton and the end of this walk.

Walk 4: Russian Hill

🏢 🛒 ✕ 📷

General location: In northeastern San Francisco, north of downtown, west of North Beach, and south of Fisherman's Wharf

Special attractions: Restaurants and shopping; urban landscapes with varied architecture; views of the city and the bay; public art; parks

Difficulty: Strenuous, with steep hills and sets of stairs

Distance: 3.9 miles

Estimated time: 2.5 hours

Services: Restaurants, hotels, restrooms

Restrictions: Not wheelchair accessible. Dogs must be leashed and their droppings picked up.

For more information: The San Francisco Travel Association, 900 Market St., Hallidie Plaza, San Francisco, CA 94102-2804; (415) 391-2000; sanfrancisco.travel

Getting started: This walk begins at Washington Square in North Beach, at the intersection of Columbus Avenue and Union Street. GPS: N37 48.025' / W122 24.600'

(1) From the intersection of Market, Third, Kearny, and Geary Streets, go north 9.5 blocks on Kearny to Columbus. Turn left onto Columbus Avenue and go 4.5 blocks to the corner of Columbus and Union Street.

(2) From the Golden Gate Bridge, continue south on US 101 / Presidio Parkway, staying right onto Lombard Street. Drive about 1 mile on Lombard Street to Van Ness Avenue. Stay in the far left lane on Lombard, cross Van Ness, and continue on Lombard for 1 block to Polk

Street. Turn right onto Polk and go 3 blocks. Turn left on Union Street and go 7.5 blocks to the corner of Union and Columbus Avenue.

On-street parking in this neighborhood is scarce and time restricted. The small lots and garages are expensive; one of the more reasonable is the Vallejo Street Garage at 766 Vallejo. Parking is also available in nearby Chinatown at the Portsmouth Square Garage, on Kearny between Washington and Clay Streets. Using public transportation to get to Washington Square is highly recommended.

Public transportation: Several San Francisco Municipal Railway (Muni) buses stop on Washington Square near the starting point of this walk. Contact Muni for information about schedules, fares, and accessibility (sfmta.com, trip planner.transit.511.org).

Overview: Russian Hill is one of San Francisco's finest residential neighborhoods. As you wander its steep, beautifully landscaped stairways and streets, you will pass a cluster of homes that survived the 1906 earthquake and fire, and visit magical Macondray Lane, a parklike pedestrian alley. A side trip into the San Francisco Art Institute adds to the charm, offering up a mural by famed Mexican painter Diego Rivera and sweeping views from Zellerbach Quadrangle. Wind down a block of quirky Lombard Street, the famous series of brick-paved switchbacks that is one of the most popular attractions of the City by the Bay. For all its charms and attractions, this exploration of Russian Hill is not for the faint of lung or leg.

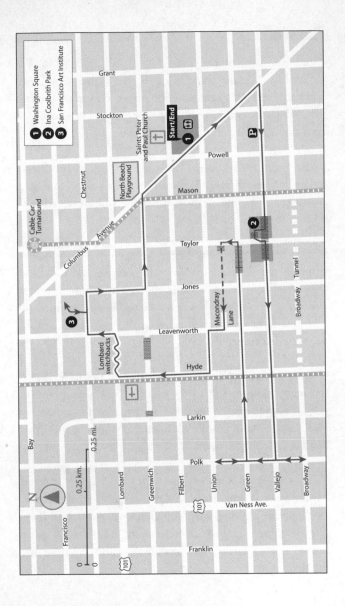

Grant

Stockton

Powell

Chestnut

Mason

Cable Car
Turnaround

Columbus   Avenue

Taylor

Jones

Leavenworth

Hyde

Larkin

Bay

Lombard

Greenwich

Filbert

Union

Green

Vallejo

Broadway

Van Ness Ave.

Franklin

Francisco

Polk

North Beach
Playground

Saints Peter
and Paul Church

Start/End

Macondray
Lane

Lombard
switchbacks

Broadway
Tunnel

1 Washington Square
2 Ina Coolbrith Park
3 San Francisco Art Institute

N

0.25 km.
0.25 mi.

0

101

The Walk

▶Start in Washington Square, at the intersection of Columbus Avenue and Union Street. Cross Columbus and then turn left to cross Union Street. Follow Columbus for 2 blocks to Vallejo Street, passing classic North Beach restaurants, pastry shops, and coffeehouses.

▶Turn right onto Vallejo. Pause for a moment and listen: Italian is spoken here. Walk a block up Vallejo and stop and listen: Chinese is spoken here, at the outer edge of Chinatown.

▶Cross Powell Street and begin the steep climb up Vallejo, entering the Russian Hill district. Pass several blocks of triple-decker flats, with their characteristic bay windows and garages underneath. Cross Mason Street and the cable car tracks; the distinctive buzzing you hear is the cables running just under the rails.

▶Reach the base of Ina Coolbrith Park at 0.5 mile, one of the many beautiful stairway parks of San Francisco. The park is named after a former California poet laureate and local literary icon. Coolbrith made her home in this once-bohemian neighborhood.

▶Take the set of stairs on the right, and climb the steep, handsomely planted hillside. Quaint cottages with patch-work gardens, along with shingled apartment buildings, line the stairs. The ornate apartment house, with pent-house, at 945 Green St. rises ahead, silhouetted against the sky.

▶At the first opportunity to leave the stairway, turn right onto the paved path that traverses the hillside, passing a set of park benches. The benches offer exceptional views of the cityscape to the east, encompassing the Bay Bridge, the Transamerica Pyramid, and the tall, dark Bank of America building.

▶Beyond the benches, mount a stone stairway that climbs straight up the hillside. At the top of these stairs, go right and then left, following the path as it switchbacks up to Taylor Street.

▶Cross Taylor Street and continue up switchbacking stairs to the balustraded overlook at the top of Russian Hill (0.8 mile). From the overlook, scanning the panorama from right to left, you'll see the rooftops of North Beach, the

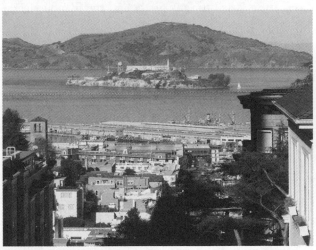

Looking north from Russian Hill, views open across the piers to Alcatraz and Angel Islands.

southern flank of Telegraph Hill, the piers at Fisherman's Wharf, and, of course, San Francisco Bay, studded with sailboats, tugs, and tankers.

▶From the summit descend along the sidewalk to the ramp at the foot of this block of Vallejo. Wonderful residences, some dating back to the early twentieth century, line the street. Take the staircase that drops briefly from the center of the ramp's headwall to Jones Street.

▶Cross Jones and continue down Vallejo past more quintessential Russian Hill flats. Cross Hyde Street and the tracks of the Powell-Hyde cable car line, which runs between Union Square and Fisherman's Wharf.

▶Walk downhill for 2 blocks (a total of 4 blocks from the Jones Street stairs) to Polk Street and the friendly neighborhood shopping district of Polk Gulch.

▶Make a short loop through this lively retail district by taking a left onto Polk, walking 1 block to Broadway, crossing Polk, and then walking back along Polk for 3 blocks to Union Street. The street is lined with wine shops, ethnic restaurants, coffeehouses, fancy grocery stores, antique shops, boutiques, and bookstores.

▶At Union take a right across Polk and then make another right, following Polk for 1 block to the corner of Green. Turn left onto Green, and walk uphill for 2 blocks to Hyde.

▶Cross Hyde and continue on Green for another 2 blocks to Jones Street. In the 1000 block of Green, between

Leavenworth and Jones Streets, you will pass some of Russian Hill's oldest homes. Remarkably, this area escaped destruction during the 1906 earthquake and fire. The octagonal house at 1067 Green was built in 1857, and the houses at 1045 and 1055 Green were built in 1866 and the 1880s, respectively. The flats at 1039–1043 Green, also built in the 1880s, were moved here after the fire. Another intriguing structure is the former firehouse at 1088 Green, built in 1907. These are private homes; please respect the owners' privacy.

▶Beyond Jones walk a partial block on Green to another overlook offering great views of the Embarcadero, North Beach, and the Financial District (2.1 miles). To the left of the overlook, descend a steep set of stairs to Taylor Street.

▶Turn left onto Taylor. Descend for a short half block to the inconspicuous wooden staircase that marks the entrance to Macondray Lane.

▶Climb the Macondray Lane stairs and enter a secretive enclave of country charm. The surface of the lane is composed of cobblestone, brick, and concrete pathways, passing between meticulously maintained vintage and modern homes. Ferns, eucalyptus, and fuchsia create a peaceful, grottolike atmosphere in one of San Francisco's most densely populated neighborhoods.

▶Cross Jones and walk another block on Macondray Lane, this one not so charming, to Leavenworth.

▶Turn right onto Leavenworth and walk half a block to Union.

▶Take a left onto Union and walk 1 block to Hyde. The original Swensen's Ice Cream parlor, a Russian Hill landmark, occupies a corner of this intersection. Ice cream cone in hand, take a right onto Hyde and walk 3 blocks to Lombard Street.

▶Turn right onto Lombard and walk down the sidewalk/ staircase that borders the bricked switchbacks of postcard fame. Undoubtedly San Francisco's most famous street, the Lombard switchbacks were installed in the 1920s to lessen the steepness of the grade for automobiles.

▶At the bottom of the switchbacks, shimmy through the crowds of camera-bearing sightseers, turn left onto Leavenworth, and walk 1 block. Alcatraz Island, once a prison and now part of the Golden Gate National Recreation Area, rises from the bay directly ahead.

▶Turn right onto Chestnut. Midway down the block, on the left (north) side of the street, enter the building that looks like a Spanish monastery. This is the San Francisco Art Institute, the city's acclaimed art school. Walk through the courtyard, passing the fountain on the left. At the far left of the courtyard, stop in the Diego Rivera Gallery to view the fresco, which depicts the "design and construction of a modern industrial city." The fresco was painted by the great Mexican muralist in 1931.

▸Exit the Rivera Gallery and continue down the corridor, away from the courtyard, to the Zellerbach Quadrangle. An addition to the historic Mission-style structure, the plaza is nautical in feel, with smokestack-like skylights that look down into the institute's studios and stark lines in gray that evoke wood bleached by sun and sea. The quadrangle opens onto some of the best views in the city, stretching from Telegraph Hill and the Bay Bridge north and west to Fisherman's Wharf.

▸Leave the art institute as you entered, exiting onto Chestnut, and turn left. Continue downhill for one-half block.

▸Turn right onto Jones Street and walk 2 blocks.

▸Turn left onto Greenwich and walk 2 blocks to Columbus Avenue, abandoning the relative tranquillity of Russian Hill for coffee-fueled North Beach.

▸Cross the cable car tracks and turn right onto Columbus. Walk 2 blocks to the corner of Columbus and Union, Washington Square, and the end of the walk.

ALONG THE BAY

Walk 5: The Embarcadero

♿🏢👪🛒✕📷

General location: On the bayside waterfront in northeastern San Francisco, just north of the Bay Bridge

Special attractions: Cafes and restaurants; bay and city views; access to ferries and bay cruises; historic district; shopping arcades and a farmers' market; the Exploratorium

Difficulty: Easy, flat, and entirely on sidewalks

Distance: 3.0 miles

Estimated time: 1.5 hours

Services: Restaurants, ferries, shopping, restrooms

Restrictions: Wheelchair accessible. Dogs must be leashed and their droppings picked up.

For more information: The San Francisco Travel Association, 900 Market St., Hallidie Plaza, San Francisco, CA 94102-2804; (415) 391-2000; sanfrancisco.travel

Getting started: This walk begins at the Ferry Building, located just north of the Bay Bridge where Market Street meets the Embarcadero. GPS: N37 47.666' / W122 23.561'

(1) From I-80 westbound take the Fremont Street exit and proceed to the intersection of Market, Fremont, and Front Streets. Cross Market and drive 3.5 blocks on Front Street to Clay Street. Turn right onto Clay and go 2 blocks to Drumm Street. Turn right onto Drumm and

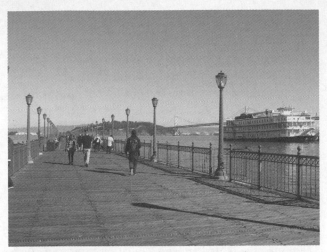

The Bay Trail public promenade stretches over the water at Pier 7.

then make a left-hand turn into the garage beneath Four Embarcadero Center.

(2) From US 101 or I-280 northbound, proceed to the intersection of Market, Third, Kearny, and Geary Streets. Drive 7 blocks on Kearny to Clay Street. Turn right onto Clay and go 6 blocks. Turn right onto Drumm and then make a left-hand turn into the garage underneath Four Embarcadero Center.

(3) From the Golden Gate Bridge, follow US 101 / Presidio Parkway south to the Marina exit, staying in the left-hand lanes as you leave the bridge. Follow Marina Boulevard and then Bay Street (a total of about 14 blocks, paralleling the bayfront to and then around Fort Mason) to the intersection of Bay and Van Ness Avenue. Continue east on Bay for 11 more blocks to the Embarcadero. Turn right onto the Embarcadero, and drive about 1 mile.

Turn right onto Washington Street and go 1 long block to Drumm Street. Turn left onto Drumm and go 1 block. Just after crossing Clay Street, make a left-hand turn into the garage underneath Four Embarcadero Center.

After parking walk through Four Embarcadero Center at street level and continue through Justin Herman Plaza to the Embarcadero. Cross the Embarcadero to reach the front of the Ferry Building.

Note: Parking is a challenge along the waterfront and in the downtown area—even the lots for the Embarcadero Center can fill up. Weekend parking may be easier to find; on weekdays many downtown lots are full by 8 a.m. The garages beneath Embarcadero Center contain more than 2,000 spaces and are free with validation from some merchants in the Embarcadero Center. You can also stow your vehicle in a less crowded garage a bit farther away from Embarcadero Center. These include:

- Fifth & Mission / Yerba Buena Gardens Garage at Fifth and Mission Streets. From the garage walk 1 block north on Fifth to Market Street and catch a Muni bus down Market to the Ferry Building. Muni Metro lines run underneath Market and connect the Powell Street Station to the Embarcadero Station near the Ferry Building.

- Portsmouth Square Garage on Kearny Street between Clay and Washington Streets. From the garage walk downhill on Clay 6 blocks. Turn right onto Drumm Street, then turn left into Four Embarcadero Center, and walk through Embarcadero Center to Justin

Herman Plaza. The Ferry Building is across the busy Embarcadero.

Public transportation: All Bay Area Rapid Transit (BART) trains and San Francisco Municipal Railway (Muni) Metro lines stop at the Embarcadero Station near the Ferry Building. A number of Muni buses also stop near the Ferry Building. Golden Gate Transit bus lines and AC Transit bus lines stop at the Transbay Terminal. Contact Muni for information about schedules, fares, and accessibility (sfmta.com, tripplanner.transit.511.org).

Overview: The Embarcadero was once a working-class thoroughfare, an industrial stretch frequented mostly by longshoremen and commuters into downtown. My grandfather, a Mexican immigrant who worked in the sugar industry, used to walk down to the waterfront from the family home on Potrero Hill after he retired, seeking the company of fellow laborers. In those days the piers were ramshackle and boarded up, the smells of the sea and tobacco smoke and machinery clinging to the buildings like they did to Tata's plaid flannel shirts.

These days the Embarcadero teems with tourists, while resident San Franciscans use the long stretch of open sidewalk to run and exercise their pets. The piers have been refurbished and repurposed, housing restaurants and businesses, tony retail outlets and art exhibitions. Street vendors and performers set up stands and stages along the sidewalk, attracting crowds that clot the thoroughfare. A pair of piers served as venues for the 2013 America's Cup races, a legacy sure to linger. The Exploratorium, the amazing hands-on science museum that once resided at the Palace of Fine Arts near the Presidio, has taken up residence at Pier 15, opening up a parklike space that invites families to linger and play along the waterfront. Openings behind the piers lead onto boardwalks on the water, including the Bay Trail public promenade, its lamp-lined wooden planks leading out onto the bay. A few of the piers remain devoted to their original use as dockside warehouses. But my grandfather would be stunned and amazed by the transformation.

The Embarcadero is a wonderful place to walk on a foggy morning. Somehow the fog makes the scene more maritime, more evocative of San Francisco's waterfront past: Foghorns sound in the distance, ghost ships slide silently by, the chop—sometimes invisible—slaps against the piers, and the salted breeze moistens your face. Be sure to check out the series of historical markers, which provide a sense of what the waterfront was like from the days of the clipper ships to the early twentieth century. Also watch for the brief, vivid poems, many of them Japanese haiku, inscribed in the pavement underfoot.

From the waterfront park that separates the Embarcadero from Fisherman's Wharf, the walk heads inland to San Francisco's first historic district, the Jackson Square neighborhood, with its antiques shops and interior design studios. By a fluke, many of the structures here—including some built in the 1850s—survived the 1906 earthquake and fire.

The Embarcadero walk culminates, appropriately enough, in the Embarcadero Center, an upscale shopping-and-dining complex extending over 8 city blocks. The center stands just opposite the Ferry Building where the walk begins.

The Walk

►Start at the front entrance to the Ferry Building, below the clock tower. Ferries bound for the Marin County cities of Larkspur and Sausalito depart from the Ferry Building. But that's not its main attraction: It now serves as a marketplace for local cheesemakers, bakers, sausage makers, coffee roasters, and chocolatiers, among others. On Tuesday, Thursday, and Saturday, a farmers' market stretches in front of the building and beyond, with vendors selling locally grown produce, handmade jams, preserves, and relishes, and other foodstuffs. Stands selling prepared dishes occupy one end of the market—it smells like heaven.

►As you face the Ferry Building, odd-numbered piers run to the left, even numbers to the right. Turn left and begin walking on the esplanade past Pier 1, home of the Port of San Francisco (sfport.com) and departure point for the San Francisco Ferry to Alameda, Oakland, and other points east and north. The skyscrapers of the Financial District rise to the left as you walk along the esplanade.

►The Bay Trail public promenade is at Pier 7, near the intersection of Broadway and the Embarcadero. This long boardwalk, lined with old-fashioned street lamps, extends out into the bay. Stroll to the end of the pier to feel the bay breezes, get a closer view of sailboats and ferries as they pass, and watch anglers try their luck.

From Pier 7 you can look south to the ferryboat *Santa Rosa*, permanently docked at Pier 3, and enjoy great views of the Bay Bridge and Treasure Island. The Transamerica Pyramid, a signature feature of the San Francisco skyline,

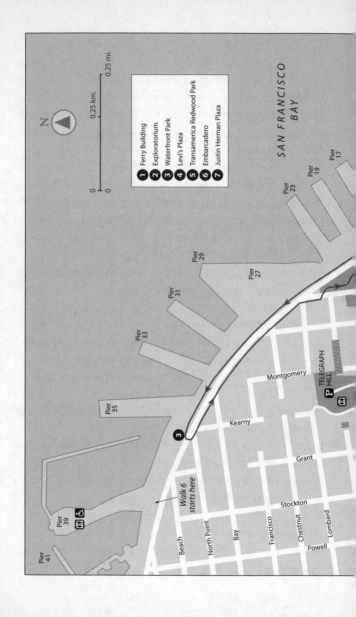

N

0   0.25 km.
0   0.25 mi.

1 Ferry Building
2 Exploratorium
3 Waterfront Park
4 Levi's Plaza
5 Transamerica Redwood Park
6 Embarcadero
7 Justin Herman Plaza

SAN FRANCISCO BAY

Pier 41
Pier 39
Pier 35
Pier 33
Pier 31
Pier 29
Pier 27
Pier 23
Pier 19
Pier 17

Montgomery
TELEGRAPH HILL
Kearny
Grant
Stockton
Beach
North Point
Bay
Francisco
Chestnut
Lombard
Powell

Walk 6 starts here

3

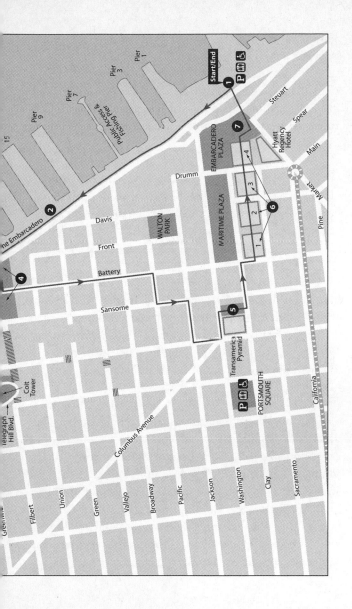

Start/End

Pier 1

Pier 3

Pier 7

Pier 9

Public Access & Fishing Pier

15

The Embarcadero

Steuart

Spear

Main

Market

Pine

California

Sacramento

Clay

Washington

Jackson

Pacific

Broadway

Vallejo

Green

Union

Filbert

Greenwich

Columbus Avenue

Davis

Front

Battery

Sansome

Drumm

WALTON PARK

EMBARCADERO PLAZA

MARITIME PLAZA

Hyatt Regency Hotel

Transamerica Pyramid

PORTSMOUTH SQUARE

Coit Tower

Telegraph Hill Blvd.

dominates the skyline as you walk west, back to the esplanade.

▶Pass the Exploratorium at Piers 15–17 (0.6 mile). Look at the skyline for a good view of Telegraph Hill, with Coit Tower at its peak and homes perched precariously on its steep slopes.

▶Pass Piers 19–23, which served as the venue for America's Cup races in 2013. Pier 27 was slated to open as San Francisco's new cruise terminal as of 2014, and the development includes a 2.5-acre park called Northeast Wharf Plaza.

▶When you are opposite Pier 23, cross the Embarcadero at the crosswalk to see a small historical marker with photos of the White Angel Jungle, a Depression-era soup kitchen that stood nearby. Here Lois Jordan, the "White Angel," fed "seamen without ships, longshoremen with no cargo to load, railroad men out of jobs, carpenters with nothing to build."

▶Levi's Plaza is next door to the White Angel marker. This small park is adjacent to the corporate headquarters of Levi Strauss & Co., the well-known jeans-manufacturing company founded in 1873. Beyond the park, in the Levi Strauss office complex, are several restaurants and a large fountain, its waters cascading over granite and concrete ledges. The lobby of the glass-fronted main building of Levi Strauss & Co. features a display that recounts the company's colorful history.

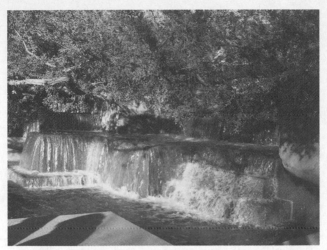
Levi's Plaza, just off the Embarcadero, packs lawn, shade trees, and a fountain into a small space.

▶Exit Levi's Plaza where you entered it, cross back onto the Embarcadero, and turn left to continue your ramble around the eastern tip of the San Francisco Peninsula. A little farther on, the last tall historic marker commemorates the old North Point–Lombard & Greenwich dock, the destination for clipper ships that rounded Cape Horn in the 1850s and 1860s. From this vantage point the side of Telegraph Hill looks scooped out . . . and, in fact, it was. Ships would unload their cargo in San Francisco, fill their holds with Telegraph Hill rock for ballast, and then head back around the cape.

▶Pass Pier 33, where ferries depart for Alcatraz Island.

▶Continue on the esplanade toward the stand of colorful flags that marks the beginning of Waterfront Park, which extends from Pier 35 to Pier 41 (1.25 miles). This broad expanse of boardwalk features benches from which you can gaze across the bay at Angel Island and the Richmond–San Rafael Bridge in the distance, and listen to the bay waters lapping against the piers. Other seating areas are set off by cobblestone paving stones and well-tended plantings— ideal for a picnic or a breather. PIER 39, a bonanza of shopping and restaurants, is at the other end of the park, if you're hungry.

▶Return to the flagpoles at the beginning of Waterfront Park. Cross the Embarcadero at the crosswalk, turn left, and walk 3 blocks to the intersection with Battery and Lombard Streets.

▶Cross to the opposite corner of Battery, where you'll find the Fog City restaurant. This restaurant once was a classic diner, from the shiny chrome dining-car exterior to the diner staples served inside. As of 2013 the diner's gone upscale, like the piers across the street, resurfaced in wood and glass and serving fancy cocktails and specialties like Berkshire pork cheeks and Kampachi crudo. An old brick warehouse building rises across the street from Fog City, at 1333 Battery, handsome arched windows looking down on the Embarcadero from several floors up.

▶Walk down Battery to the entrance of Levi's Plaza. Turn left into the park and follow the curved path through the park. After passing the small fountain with water tumbling over different levels, turn right and walk back to Battery Street.

▶Turn left onto Battery and go 5 blocks to Pacific Avenue.

▶Turn right onto Pacific and walk 1 block to Sansome Street. Cross Sansome, and then cross Pacific.

▶Go 1 block on Sansome to Jackson Street. Notice the distinctive building facades at 710 and 712 Sansome.

▶Turn right onto Jackson and walk 1 block along this charming tree-lined street, at the heart of the Jackson Square Historic District, which hosts fine antiques stores, decorator shops, and oriental rug and vintage poster dealers. This neighborhood also escaped the 1906 fire and offers a rare glimpse into gold rush–era San Francisco in its ornate facades, constructed of stone and cast iron. Especially notable is the Hotaling Building, originally home to a wholesale liquor company, at 451 Jackson.

▶Turn left onto Montgomery Street and walk 1 block to Washington Street. The historic Belli Building, at 722–728 Montgomery, once held the law offices of famed criminal defense attorney Melvin Belli. Built in 1851, it is believed to be the oldest surviving building in downtown San Francisco. This structure was also known as the Genella Building, after original owner Joseph Genella, purveyor of glassware and fine china. It was home to many artists' studios between the 1880s and the 1930s.

▶Cross Washington and enter the lobby of the Transamerica Pyramid. Wheelchair-accessible doors are located on the Washington Street side of this corner of the pyramid. Walk through the lobby, which features art exhibitions, to the virtual observation deck. Here, four screens show views—transmitted from scopes mounted on top of the pyramid—to the north, south, east, and west. Feel free to move a scope's orientation and zoom in to see all quadrants of San Francisco—in real time and astonishing detail. Kids will love it.

▸Exit the Transamerica Pyramid the same way you entered it and go right on Washington for one-half block to the entrance of Transamerica Redwood Park. Turn right and walk through the park to the opposite entrance on Clay Street, just beyond the "frog pond" fountain. This park's solemn redwoods—transplanted from the Santa Cruz mountains—along with its flowers, greenery, and whimsical bronze sculptures, create a breathing space at the edge of the Financial District.

▸Exit the park onto Clay and turn left. Go 1.5 blocks to Battery Street. Pass a bronze plaque that marks a site linking today's Financial District to its mercantile past near the corner of Clay and Sansome Streets. During the gold rush, when San Francisco's shoreline came up to Montgomery Street, the ship *Niantic* graced this location; no longer a seafaring vessel, it was used instead as offices, stores, and a warehouse in the fast-growing young city.

▸Cross Clay, cross Battery, and proceed a partial block on Battery to the entrance of One Embarcadero Center. A ramp for wheelchairs is located on the right side of the entrance area.

Embarcadero Center fills 4 square city blocks. The lower three levels of its four office towers are home to scores of shops and restaurants. Escalators are positioned at the center of each building, and wheelchair-accessible elevators are located adjacent to the elevators to the parking garages. Wheelchair-accessible restrooms are located on the lobby level of each building.

▶Walk through One Embarcadero Center toward its exit on Front Street, following signs to Two Embarcadero Center. Continue walking through the shopping complex, following signs to Three Embarcadero Center and Four Embarcadero Center.

▶Exit Four Embarcadero Center onto Justin Herman Plaza, a well-loved open space. On warm days people relax near the fountain or at the sidewalk tables on the terrace. During the summer Embarcadero Center hosts outdoor concerts. Street merchants do a brisk business on the Market Street side of the plaza, especially during the holiday season. Justin Herman Plaza also is home to two public sculptures. The *Vaillancourt Fountain* dominates the landscape at the north end of the plaza. Created by Montreal sculptor Armand Vaillancourt, the fountain is made up of 101 boxes of precast aggregate concrete. At the other end of the plaza, near the Hyatt Regency, check out the bright metal sculpture called *La Chiffonnière*. Created by French artist Jean Dubuffet, *La Chiffonnière* ("Rag Woman") is constructed of stainless steel with linear tracings of black epoxy.

▶Cross the Embarcadero to the Ferry Building and the end of this walk.

Walk 6: Fisherman's Wharf

♿🏢👪🛒🍽📷

General location: On the bay waterfront in northeastern San Francisco, just north of North Beach and Russian Hill

Special attractions: Museums and an aquarium; the PIER 39 shopping arcade; cafes and restaurants, coastline views; a floating national historic park; sea lion viewing; access to ferries and bay cruises

Difficulty: Easy, flat, and entirely on sidewalks

Distance: 3.5 miles

Estimated time: 2 hours

Services: Parking, restaurants, restrooms

Restrictions: Wheelchair accessible. Dogs must be leashed and their droppings picked up.

For more information: The San Francisco Travel Association, 900 Market St., Hallidie Plaza, San Francisco, CA 94102-2804; (415) 391-2000; sanfrancisco.travel

Getting started: This walk begins at Waterfront Park near PIER 39, on the Embarcadero opposite Beach Street. GPS: N37 48.466'/W122 24.457'

(1) From I-80 westbound take the Harrison Street/Embarcadero exit—the first left exit after crossing the Bay Bridge. Turn right onto Harrison Street, go 4 blocks, then turn left onto the Embarcadero and continue about 1.5 miles to PIER 39.

(2) From the San Francisco Peninsula, take US 101 north to I-80 eastbound. Take the Fourth Street exit and go east on Bryant Street almost 1 mile. Turn left onto the Embarcadero and continue almost 2 miles to PIER 39.

You can also take I-280 north to the Sixth Street exit, then follow Bryant and the Embarcadero to PIER 39.

(3) From the Golden Gate Bridge, follow US 101 / Presidio Parkway south to the Marina exit, staying in the left-hand lanes as you leave the bridge. Follow Marina Boulevard and then Bay Street (a total of about 14 blocks, paralleling the bayfront to and then around Fort Mason) to the intersection of Bay and Van Ness Avenue. Continue on Bay for 11 blocks, turn left onto the Embarcadero, and go 2.5 blocks to PIER 39.

On-street parking is extremely difficult in the Fisherman's Wharf area, and parking garages are quite expensive. Parking is available at the PIER 39 Garage directly across the Embarcadero from PIER 39; at the Anchorage shopping center on Jones Street between Beach and North Point Streets; at Ghirardelli Square, on Beach between Polk and Larkin Streets; and at numerous street-level parking lots in the area. These parking garages have wheelchair-accessible parking areas.

Note: To avoid Fisherman's Wharf congestion, you may prefer to park in the lots at Fort Mason Center or along the Marina Green, and do the walk in reverse, starting at the Municipal Pier in Aquatic Park and turning around at PIER 39. To reach the Municipal Pier from the Fort Mason Center, climb the steep stairs (not wheelchair accessible) leading out of the Fort Mason Center parking lot opposite Building E. At the top turn left and take the brief, delightful walk along the paved path as it rounds the hilly headland between Fort Mason Center and Aquatic Park, then descends to the pier.

Public transportation: San Francisco Municipal Railway (Muni) runs buses from the downtown area to within a few blocks of PIER 39, as well as to Aquatic Park. Both the Powell/Hyde and Powell/Mason cable car lines run to the Fisherman's Wharf area. Contact Muni for information about schedules, fares, and accessibility (sfmta.com, tripplanner.transit.511.org).

Overview: Fisherman's Wharf is among the top destinations for visitors to San Francisco—and with good reason. The wharf stretches from carnival-like PIER 39 to the curving municipal pier at Aquatic Park. A host of attractions lie between: the Hyde Street Pier, a floating national park that is home to a collection of historic ships; a vast number of eateries, many serving seafood caught fresh that day; the shopping meccas known as the Cannery and Ghirardelli Square, housed in old brick factories; and the fascinating San Francisco Maritime Museum.

Though this walk is not particularly long or strenuous, allow plenty of time to explore, have a meal, and do some shopping. An early-morning start is also recommended: the wharves are less crowded then and the fog will likely not have burned off, adding a dash of romance to the often bustling scene.

Fisherman's Wharf remains the home of San Francisco's commercial and sport fishing fleets, as it has been since the turn of the twentieth century. But the fishing industry is much smaller than in years past, with fisheries restricted if decreased fish and/or crab populations can't support the fleet. Tourism is the real business of Fisherman's Wharf, with the PIER 39, Cannery, and Ghirardelli shopping and dining arcades a powerful draw. Still, the attractions that celebrate San Francisco's seagoing past, like the floating museum at Hyde Street Pier and the San Francisco Maritime Museum in Aquatic Park, are well worth visiting. And the Municipal Pier is the perfect escape from the tourist frenzy. Walk out to the end, take a deep breath, gaze out across the bay, and imagine the days when fishing boats, clipper ships, paddle tugs, and schooners swarmed these fabled waters.

The Walk

▸Start in Waterfront Park, gazing out at the sailboats and fishing vessels moored in the Pier 39 Marina. Follow the Embarcadero through a linear open space outfitted with benches and planters thick with blooms.

▸Reach PIER 39 and turn right into the main entrance. The sidewalk in front of the entrance is often congested, as street vendors and performers set up shop, hoping for a generous share of the attention of passersby. Follow the crowds through the mall, visiting shops, restaurants, and the carousel. A second level offers more tantalizing opportunities for the hungry and the gift-seeker. The pier also is home to the Aquarium of the Bay, which offers close encounters with sea life behind glass. An expansive view of San Francisco Bay opens at the end of the pier, including Alcatraz Island with Angel Island behind it, Treasure and Yerba Buena Islands, and the Bay Bridge. On any day you'll see an array of seagoing vessels, from kayaks to sailboats, barges to tugboats, cruise ships to ferries. Stop for a moment, watch, and marvel.

▸Continue around the end of PIER 39, and bearing left, walk along the railing on the west side of the PIER 39 complex. Here you will find a noisy pride of sea lions—as

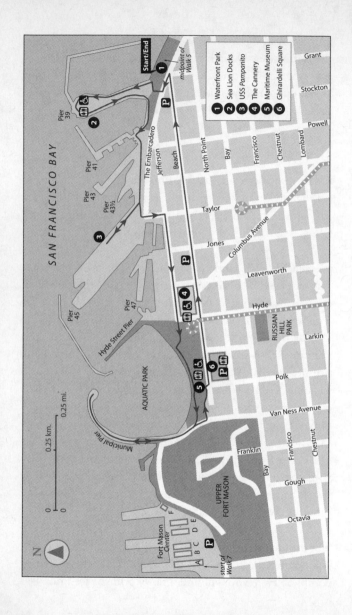

Start/End
1

midpoint of Walk 5

1 Waterfront Park
2 Sea Lion Docks
3 USS *Pampanito*
4 The Cannery
5 Maritime Museum
6 Ghirardelli Square

1
2
3
4
5
6

Grant
Stockton
Powell
Lombard
Chestnut
Francisco
Bay
North Point
Jefferson
Beach
The Embarcadero

Pier 39
Pier 41
Pier 43
Pier 43½
Pier 45
Pier 47
Hyde Street Pier

SAN FRANCISCO BAY

Taylor
Jones
Leavenworth
Hyde
Larkin
Polk
Van Ness Avenue
Franklin
Gough
Octavia

Columbus Avenue

RUSSIAN HILL PARK

AQUATIC PARK

Municipal Pier

Chestnut
Bay
Francisco

UPPER FORT MASON

Fort Mason Center

start of Walk 7

A B C D E F

0.25 mi.
0.25 km.

N

many as 200 of them—lolling on old wooden docks. You can hear them barking before you round the corner, and you will certainly smell them. The sea lions of Fisherman's Wharf are a riot to watch, jostling each other for a place in the sun.

▶Continue along PIER 39's perimeter, walking back toward the Embarcadero. At the first opportunity turn right and walk alongside the railing at the docks of the Blue & Gold tour-boat and ferry fleet.

▶Just beyond the Blue & Gold fleet harbor, turn right and walk on the lamppost-lined boardwalk that stretches out into the bay at Pier 41. A 12-foot-square relief map showing the bay, the San Francisco Peninsula, the East Bay, and the North Bay can be found in a seating area on the right side of the boardwalk, in what looks like a large planter.

▶Return down the boardwalk, turn right, and walk past the terminal for the ferries to Alcatraz Island and Angel Island, as well as for several bay tour boats.

▶Just beyond Pier 41, walk out on the wooden surface of an aborted continuation of the Embarcadero. An archway like those found on the piers south of Waterfront Park frames views of historic ships available for touring on Pier 45.

▶Walk out on Pier 45 to view the USS *Pampanito*, a World War II fleet submarine open for touring. As you walk along the pier, note the signs—surely unique in a tourist area—that warn you not to sit on the torpedoes alongside the wharf building. The SS *Jeremiah O'Brien*, a Liberty ship, is moored behind the *Pampanito*; this "living museum," which is listed on the National Register of Historic Places and is a National Historic Landmark, is also available for touring. The Musée Mecanique, an amazing collection of historic arcade games, is housed on Pier 45 as well.

▶Turn right once you leave the pier, and walk about 100 feet to the intersection of Taylor Street and the end of the Embarcadero.

▶Turn left to cross the Embarcadero, and follow Taylor 1 short block to Jefferson Street. On the right side of Taylor, colorful outdoor stalls sell whole crabs as well as seafood cocktails that you can savor as you walk along.

▶Turn right onto Jefferson and walk 2 blocks to Leavenworth Street. On your right you will pass the Jefferson Street lagoon, where commercial fishing boats dock after selling their catch. These tightly packed docks are a jumble of white boats trimmed in cheerful tones of green, blue, yellow, and red. Most are weatherworn, and a few appear barely seaworthy. This appealing harbor is lined with seafood restaurants, with picture windows that open onto the bay, and a plethora of gift shops.

▶At the corner of Jefferson and Leavenworth, cross Jefferson and turn right. As you continue through this more crowded section of Fisherman's Wharf, keep an eye out for the notorious "Bushman." For more than 30 years, according to sfgate.com, one (or two) of San Francisco's

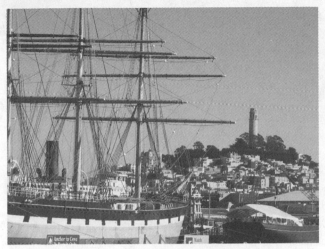

The end of the Municipal Pier, which curls around Aquatic Park, affords views of Coit Tower framed by the masts of the tall ship *Balclutha*.

most persistent street performers, costumed in leafy twigs, has crouched at the edge of the sidewalk, looking like a decorative bush. When an unwary tourist passes, Bush-man leaps up, throws out his arms, and scares the daylights out of his target. Amused onlookers gather some distance away, watching this scene unfold again and again.

▶Reach the Cannery, an old brick building, once a Del Monte packing plant, which now houses restaurants and stores. The Cannery's street-level courtyard is quite pleas-ant, planted with olive trees and other non-leaping shrubs.

▶After exploring the Cannery, exit onto Jefferson Street and walk to the end of the block at Hyde Street.

A FLOATING MUSEUM

From a side-wheel ferry to a scow schooner, a square-rigged sailing vessel to steam-driven tugs, the "floating museum" officially known as the San Francisco Maritime National Historical Park is a must-see attraction along Fisherman's Wharf.

Walk out on the Hyde Street Pier to visit the historic ships that make this park unique. Here you will find the towering three-masted sailing ship *Balclutha*; a pair of oceangoing tugs, *Eppleton Hall* and *Hercules*; the last San Francisco Bay scow schooner still floating, *Alma*; the *Eureka*, a powerful early twentieth-century ferry; and a schooner used in the lumbering trade, *C. A. Thayer*.

The three largest vessels—the *Balclutha, Eureka,* and *C. A. Thayer*—are open for touring; you can walk the decks and peek into the cabins and holds. Sailors and shipwrights regularly demonstrate seafaring skills here, and the many excellent exhibits document more than a century of San Francisco waterfront history. The *Balclutha* also hosts overnight field trips for Bay Area students, re-creating with sometimes frightening (for a fifth grader) accuracy life as a greenhorn on a tall ship in the gold-rush era. From remembering to hail the captain for permission to come aboard to peeling potatoes in the tiny galley and launching a longboat, students leave the ship with memories that last a lifetime.

The San Francisco Maritime Museum, at the foot of Polk Street, is a key part of this maritime national park. The museum features the Steamship Room, nautical artifacts, and special exhibits on whaling, the China trade, and the days of the gold rush, when scores of captains and crews abandoned their ships in San Francisco harbor and headed for the goldfields. You may also want to stop in at the Maritime Research Center/J. Porter Shaw Library at Fort Mason Center, Building E. It features 12,000 volumes on maritime subjects.

For those who want to learn even more, the national park regularly offers classes, talks, demonstrations, and tours. Learn about battleships, pirates, and the crafting of wooden boats. And if you love the music of the sea, the park sponsors monthly concerts that feature ballads, sailor's songs, chanteys, and nautical fiddle airs. For more information, visit nps.gov/safr.

►Turn right and cross Jefferson. Straight ahead lies the Hyde Street Pier, home to the "floating" San Francisco Maritime National Historical Park. Take some time to visit this intriguing collection of historic ships, and the wonderful bookstore featuring an abundance of nautical tomes.

►Turn left onto Jefferson to enter Aquatic Park, a bustling public space that includes Victorian Park (designed by famed landscape architect Thomas Church), the San Francisco Maritime Museum, the Hyde Street cable car turnaround, and a curving municipal pier that embraces the quiet cove.

As you enter Aquatic Park, note the two old buildings on your right. These are the clubhouses of two legendary swimming and boating clubs that date back before the turn of the twentieth century: the South End Rowing Club and the Dolphin Club. Club members swim year-round in the bracing waters of Aquatic Park. If you spot a bright-orange swim cap bobbing in the water, you have seen a club swimmer at work/play.

▶Staying close to the water, follow the promenade around the cove, tracing the curve of a sandy beach. A set of concrete bleachers faces the cove, and the San Francisco Maritime Museum rises above. This artistic Streamline Moderne building was modeled after an ocean liner of the 1930s.

▶At the west end of the cove, take the asphalt ramp that slopes gently up and away from the water toward the quiet, tree-lined ending of Van Ness Avenue, which is a congested thoroughfare just a couple of blocks to the south.

▶Turn right onto the sidewalk and walk 1 block to the intersection of Van Ness and McDowell Street and the beginning of the Municipal Pier (1.75 miles). Also known as the Aquatic Park Pier, it is open daily from dawn to dusk.

▶Walk out onto the pier. A great way to get out on the bay without a boat, the pier offers the best landlubber's view of Alcatraz Island, as well as splendid views of the Golden Gate Bridge and the Marin Headlands. For those strolling via wheelchair, use the wide center roadway; the lanes on either side of the roadway, created by concrete curbs, get uncomfortably narrow in a few spots, and you cannot get out of these lanes until the very end of the pier. Anglers and crabbers also set up their rigs in the lanes.

▶After your tour of the pier, walk up the sidewalk on the left side of Van Ness Avenue for about 1 block, passing the whimsically round former restroom with exterior stairs and an observation deck (closed). Continue past the gently sloping ramp that you used previously to reach Van Ness Avenue.

▶Turn left onto the next paved pathway, which is quite wide and slopes downward toward the maritime museum. A covered bocce ball court is on the right, often crowded with groups of men and women seriously engaged in this Mediterranean sport. The two tall, curving condominium towers behind the bocce ball courts are sometimes called the "Buck Teeth on the Bay."

▶Walk to the front entrance of the San Francisco Maritime Museum on Beach Street, taking the ramp that leads to the polished chrome front doors. The maritime museum is a must-see for anyone entranced by the lore of the sea. Portions of the museum's collection—ranging from models of clipper ships to actual fishing boats—are on display, and fascinating rotating exhibits focus on San Francisco's rich maritime heritage. Created as a recreation center and bathhouse by the Works Progress Administration during the 1930s, the museum features ocean-inspired murals in the lobby and cheerful mosaics of sea creatures on the balcony overlooking Aquatic Park.

▶Exit the museum through its front entrance and turn left onto Beach Street. On your right, between Polk and Larkin Streets, is another early-day factory turned shopping center. Ghirardelli Square was originally a woolen mill and then—you guessed it—a chocolate factory. Now it is packed with specialty shops, restaurants with splendid bay views, and of course, San Francisco's own Ghirardelli Chocolate shop.

▶Walk along Beach for 2 blocks to Hyde Street. Beach Street is often lined with street artists and craftspeople selling their wares. As you near Hyde, you will pass the Hyde Street cable car turnaround on your left.

▶At the corner of Beach and Hyde, cross Beach, and then cross Hyde. The Buena Vista Cafe, a San Francisco landmark, is on the southwest corner of this intersection. The cafe is known as the place where, in 1952, the first Irish coffee in America was served.

▶Continue on Beach for 7 blocks until you reach the Embarcadero at PIER 39, Waterfront Park, and the end of this walk.

Walk 7: Marina Green

♿🏢🍂👪🛒🍽

General location: Along the bay shoreline in north San Francisco, roughly equidistant between the Golden Gate Bridge and the Bay Bridge

Special attractions: Cultural attractions and restaurants at the Fort Mason Center; marinas and harbors with bay views; the one-of-a-kind Wave Organ; Palace of Fine Arts

Difficulty: Easy and flat; on sidewalks or asphalt (out to the Wave Organ)

Distance: 3.75 miles

Estimated time: 2 hours

Services: Parking, restaurants, restrooms, visitor information center. The route begins in the Golden Gate National Recreation Area (GGNRA).

Restrictions: This walk is mostly wheelchair accessible, except for the section leading out to the Wave Organ. Dogs must be leashed and their droppings picked up.

For more information: The San Francisco Travel Association, 900 Market St., Hallidie Plaza, San Francisco, CA 94102-2804; (415) 391-2000; sanfrancisco.travel. Golden Gate National Recreation Area, Fort Mason, Building 201, San Francisco, CA 94123-0022; (415) 561-4700; nps.gov/goga.

Getting started: This walk begins at the Fort Mason Center, located just west of Fisherman's Wharf and Aquatic Park. GPS: N37 48.334' / W122 25.928'

(1) From the intersection of Market, Ninth, Hayes, and Larkin Streets near the Civic Center downtown, veer

left onto Hayes and go 3 blocks. Turn right onto Franklin Street and go almost 2 miles to Bay Street. Turn left onto Bay and follow the traffic as it turns right onto Laguna Street for 2 blocks and then left onto Marina Boulevard for 1 block. At the stoplight at Beach Street, Buchanan Street, and Marina Boulevard, make a sharp right turn into the parking lot outside Fort Mason Center.

(2) From the Golden Gate Bridge, follow US 101 / Presidio Parkway south to the Marina exit, staying in the left-hand lanes of the parkway as you leave the bridge. Follow Marina Boulevard to the stoplight at Marina Boulevard and Buchanan Street. Turn left at the light and then make an immediate right into the Fort Mason Center parking lot.

There is parking—and designated wheelchair-accessible spaces—both within and just outside the Fort Mason Center gate, as well as along the Marina Green west of Fort Mason.

Public transportation: San Francisco Municipal Railway (Muni) buses stop at Fort Mason Center and at other stops within 5 or 6 blocks of Fort Mason. Contact Muni for information about schedules, fares, and accessibility (sfmta.com, tripplanner.transit.511.org).

Overview: Sailboats setting off for a jaunt around the bay, kites darting to and fro, joggers setting a brisk pace, a sea breeze caressing your face: This bayside ramble along the Marina Green makes the most of San Francisco's fabulous bayfront.

With its sweeping lawn, yacht harbors, and shoreline promenade, the Marina Green serves as both a destination for tourists and a neighborhood park for residents of the adjoining Marina District. Athletically inclined

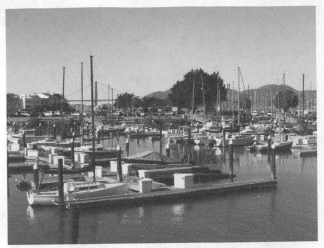

Look out over Gashouse Cove to the Golden Gate Bridge.

locals—runners, skaters, cyclists, walkers—use the green, the adjacent parcours (exercise) stations, and the adjoining GGNRA parklands as a training ground, as well as a place to lounge, picnic, toss a Frisbee, or kick a soccer ball with the kids. But it's not just for the city folk: Visitors from around the bay and elsewhere use the broad public pathways to stretch their legs and visit with their walking partners.

The walk begins at the Fort Mason Center, one of several military installations in and around San Francisco now managed by the National Park Service as part of the magnificent Golden Gate National Recreation Area. In fact, the GGNRA headquarters is housed in the center (Building 201); stop in for information about this vast urban park, one of the largest of its kind in the world. The route then follows the Marina Green to its end, where you head right to check out the one-of-a-kind Wave Organ, and left to explore the manicured grounds of the Palace of Fine Arts. Finish by strolling back along the green, savoring the salt air and watching the sailboats sway gently in their berths in East Harbor and Gashouse Cove.

Note: A walk along the Marina Green can be combined with the Golden Gate Promenade (Walk 8) for a 7-mile, leg-stretching, out-and-back ramble along the bay shoreline linking Fort Mason to Fort Point. The two walks meet at the bayside benches in the parking lot just west of the St. Francis Yacht Club.

The Walk

▶Start on the south side of Fort Mason's Building A, just inside the wall that separates Fort Mason Center from the yacht basin—called Gashouse Cove—and the parking lot outside its gate. On Sunday Fort Mason hosts a farmers' market, where locally grown produce and homemade yummies are sold. Fort Mason is also a hub for local theater and performing arts, home of the Herbst Pavilion, the Festival Pavilion, schools of music and improv, museums, art galleries, restaurants, and other attractions. Visit fort mason.org for more information.

▶Walk through the opening in Fort Mason's perimeter wall where it abuts Building A, or pass through the main gate, and descend the gentle ramp to the yacht harbor on Gashouse Cove.

▶Follow the waterside sidewalk as it curves around the perimeter of Gashouse Cove and adjoining East Harbor.

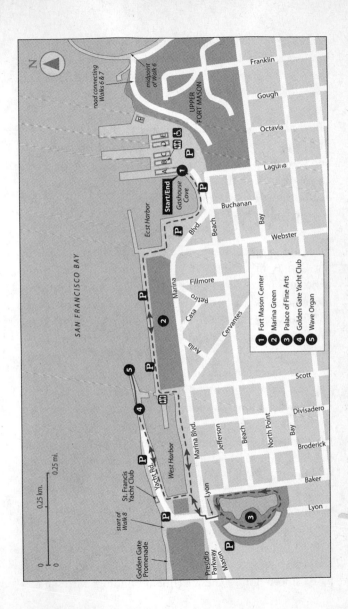

N

SAN FRANCISCO BAY

Franklin

Gough

Octavia

Laguna

Buchanan

Bay

Webster

UPPER
FORT MASON

road connecting
Walks 6 & 7

midpoint
of Walk 6

Start/End

Gashouse Cove

East Harbor

Marina Blvd.

Beach

Marina

Retiro

Casa

Cervantes

Avila

Fillmore

Scott

Divisadero

Broderick

Baker

Lyon

North Point

Bay

Beach

Jefferson

Marina Blvd.

West Harbor

Yacht Rd.

St. Francis Yacht Club

start of
Walk 8

Golden Gate
Promenade

Presidio Parkway

Mason

Lyon

0.25 km.

0.25 mi.

1 Fort Mason Center
2 Marina Green
3 Palace of Fine Arts
4 Golden Gate Yacht Club
5 Wave Organ

Sparkling white and blue sailboats rock gently in their berths, creating soft music as their lines clink against masts, the wooden docks creak, and the gulls call. The occasional boom of a foghorn punctuates the concert.

▶Beyond the harbors the route meets the Marina Green. This long swath of lawn is often crowded on weekends, and walkers, runners, cyclists, and skaters crowd the promenades that flank the green. Set out on the shoreline promenade, though you can walk along the streetside path if you prefer.

▶Pass the range house for the US Naval Magnetic Silencing Range, in the middle of the open stretch of promenade, and look out across the water. Directly opposite the range house is the jetty, or spit of land, with a little beach and the stone Wave Organ at its end. Benches line the breakwater; take a seat and join the gulls in contemplation of water, land, wind, and sky. Alcatraz Island, topped with its prison/fortress, rises in the middle of the bay. A bit farther out is the larger rise of Angel Island, and beyond that, its expensive homes sparkling white among the oaks, is the Marin County community of Tiburon. Look westward to the Golden Gate Bridge, spanning the channel separating San Francisco and Marin County, and in the middle distance, a red tile roof marks the St. Francis Yacht Club.

▶Toward the west end of the green, the promenade turns left and passes the eastern edge of West Harbor to meet Marina Boulevard. This curve allows you to check out the distinctive architecture of the Marina District, with its pastel stucco homes and apartment buildings with big bay

FORT MASON CENTER

Fort Mason Center is a "swords into plowshares" success. A military installation for more than 200 years, the site was turned over to the National Park Service in 1972 and now serves as a community and cultural center.

Fort Mason Center is home to a number of nonprofits, including museums, galleries, and theater groups. Among the organizations housed at the center are the Museo Italo Americano, the Mexican Museum, the San Francisco Museum of Modern Art's Artists Gallery, BATS Improv, Magic Theater, and the Young Performers Theater. Fort Mason Center is also home to the City College of San Francisco's Arts Campus. The headquarters for the Golden Gate National Recreation Area is also located here, in Building 201.

For the hungry, Fort Mason offers two excellent eateries: Cooks and Company in Building B for takeout sandwiches, and the renowned Greens Restaurant, in Building A overlooking Gashouse Cove, for the finest in vegetarian cuisine (greensrestaurant .com). For entertainment and even more food, check out Off the Grid's Friday night events (offthegridsf .com/markets/fort-mason-center#about).

windows and Spanish tile roofs. Built on landfill that was deposited for the Panama-Pacific International Exposition of 1915, the Marina was known as a quiet, somewhat boring residential neighborhood until the earthquake of 1989. During the quake the landfill shook like jelly and brought a few buildings to their knees. Since rebuilt, the Marina has become a trendy and expensive neighborhood.

▶Arrive on Marina Boulevard at the stoplight/intersection with Scott Street and Cervantes Boulevard. If you want to search out restaurants or boutiques, both Cervantes and Scott lead to the neighborhood shopping district on Chestnut Street, 6 blocks to the south.

▶Turn right and walk along Marina Boulevard on the boulevard promenade. This noisy stretch of roadway is a principal access route to the Golden Gate Bridge. Up ahead, a line of trees marks the end of the westward progression of this walk, and to the right (bayside), you can check out the sailboats in the West Harbor.

▶At the end of the yacht harbor, turn right and follow the broad asphalt path toward the bay and the St. Francis Yacht Club, fronted by a stand of cypress trees.

▶Cross the parking lot on the west side of the St. Francis Yacht Club to benches that overlook the bay. For those who wish to combine a stroll along the Marina Green with the Golden Gate Promenade, these bay-viewing benches mark the spot where the two walks meet.

▶To continue to the Wave Organ, return to the sidewalk adjacent to the yacht basin and continue east onto the spit. Pass the boat lift and the spot where people rinse salt water off their boats and gear. Continue along the asphalt walkway toward a miniature stone lighthouse.

▶Reach the end of the parking lot and walk to the left of the lighthouse, which, with its crenellated tower and cobbled stonework, has a European feel.

▶Follow the paved road that leads to the Golden Gate Yacht Club and the jetty beyond.

▶Pass Golden Gate Yacht Club and continue down the dirt road to the Wave Organ at the end of the jetty. Pull up a seat on a rock or bench, and listen to the waves slap against the breakwater, drink in the salty smell of the bay, and watch the boats as they pass close by. Designed by Peter Richards of the Exploratorium and constructed by stonemason and artist George Gonzales in 1986, the Wave Organ is made up of pipes that are "played" by the waves, producing music that varies with the tides and the size of the surf. Place an ear to a pipe to listen, and keep in mind that the music that emanates from this unusual instrument can't always be heard above the crash of the surf and the voices of other visitors. While you listen you can also take in the sights: Alcatraz Island lies not far distant, and Fort Mason and its yacht basin hunker on the eastern horizon. Russian Hill rises off to the right of Fort Mason, as do Telegraph Hill and Coit Tower. With water on three sides and full exposure to the wind, the Wave Organ falls just short of being on a boat on the bay.

▶Retrace your steps to the St. Francis Yacht Club and the benches overlooking the bay at the edge of the parking lot.

▶Leaving the benches behind, walk back to Marina Boulevard on the asphalt path along the edge of the yacht basin.

THE PALACE OF FINE ARTS

In 1915 San Francisco sought to ease its collective memory of the devastating 1906 earthquake and fire by throwing a world-class party. Known as the

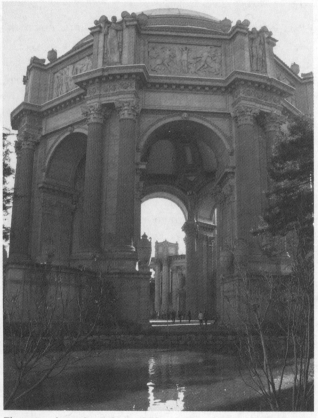

The rotunda at the Palace of Fine Arts is the last remnant of the 1915 Panama Pacific International Exposition.

Panama-Pacific International Exposition, this great fair officially celebrated the completion of the Panama Canal. For San Franciscans, however, it celebrated the rebuilding of the city and a return to normalcy.

All that remains of the grand exposition—which covered more than 600 acres, involved construction of more than one hundred buildings, and featured more than 1,500 pieces of art and sculpture—is the Palace of Fine Arts, an extravagant Beaux Arts–style structure designed by famed Bay Area architect Bernard Maybeck. Originally built of lath and plaster, the Palace—with its colonnades and rotunda—was completely restored in the 1960s.

While the rotunda and its reflecting lake have always attracted visitors, the neighboring exhibition hall was the main attraction for decades. It presently houses the Palace of Fine Arts Theater and was formerly the home of the Exploratorium, the science museum *Newsweek* has called one of the "great American amusement centers." The Exploratorium, with its hundreds of amazing hands-on exhibits, moved to Pier 15 on the Embarcadero in 2013, taking with it the delighted laughter and crowing amazement of children of all ages . . . and leaving in its wake a much quieter, contemplative palace, arguably better suited to its iconic position on the edge of a century that got off to a tumultuous start.

Turn right onto the boulevard and walk 1 short block to the light and crosswalk.

▶Cross Marina Boulevard. Take good care at this intersection: Despite the stoplights and crosswalks, drivers who continue straight ahead through the Presidio's Marina Gate on Mason Street sometimes do not stop for pedestrians, and the Presidio Parkway entrance is busy.

▶On the far side of Marina Boulevard, walk several yards to Lyon Street and the approach to the Palace of Fine Arts. A note to those in wheelchairs: There are no curb cuts allowing direct access to the Palace of Fine Arts or grounds from the sidewalk along Lyon Street. To gain access, move into the parking lot and navigate carefully to the handicapped parking area in front of the large columns to the left of the main building.

▶Turn left onto Lyon and walk 30 feet down the sidewalk, then down a short paved path and over a grassy patch to the columns next to the designated handicapped parking area.

▶Walk beneath the columns, turn left, and stroll along the pathway as it curves toward the Palace of Fine Arts park and lagoon. A number of swans ply the lagoon, and plenty of ducks and pigeons always hope for—and often receive—handfuls of broken bread from visitors. The structures invite you to gaze upward, to the carvings at the tops of the columns and the terra-cotta dome of the open pavilion. The romance of the turn-of-the-twentieth-century exposition that inspired the Palace still abides in the space. The Exploratorium, longtime resident of the exhibit hall, has moved to Pier 15 on the Embarcadero, and the building is now home to the Palace of Fine Arts Theater (palaceoffinearts.org).

▶Follow the path around the serene pond, circling back to your starting point beneath the columns at the edge of the parking lot.

▶Retrace your steps to the corner of Lyon Street and Marina Boulevard. Cross Marina Boulevard at the stoplight, turn right, and retrace your steps past West Harbor, the Marina Green, East Harbor, and Gashouse Cove to Fort Mason and the end of this walk.

Walk 8: Golden Gate Promenade

♿ 🌿 👪 📷

General location: Along the bay shoreline in north San Francisco, just east of the Golden Gate Bridge

Special attractions: Historic Fort Point; the Golden Gate Bridge; a beach, sand dunes, and tidal marsh; a municipal fishing pier; picnicking

Difficulty: Easy and flat, on crushed stone, sidewalks and asphalt

Distance: 4.0 miles

Estimated time: 2 hours

Services: Restrooms, picnic areas, visitor information center. The trail is part of the Golden Gate National Recreation Area (GGNRA).

Restrictions: The promenade is surfaced with crushed stone, a firm surface with a natural appearance. The portion of the hike on the promenade itself is handicapped accessible. While Marine Drive to Fort Point is paved, there is limited accessibility due to traffic and parking. The tour of Fort Point is not handicapped accessible.

Dogs must either be leashed or under voice control, depending on where you are walking in the GGNRA. Pets are prohibited in the marsh to protect sensitive resources. Dog droppings must be picked up. Contact the GGNRA for the most current pet regulations.

For more information: The San Francisco Travel Association, 900 Market St., Hallidie Plaza, San Francisco, CA 94102-2804; (415) 391-2000; sanfrancisco.travel. Golden Gate National Recreation Area, Fort Mason, Building

201, San Francisco, CA 94123-0022; (415) 561-4700; nps.gov/goga

Getting started: This walk begins 1 block off Marina Boulevard, just west of the St. Francis Yacht Club, near the northeast corner of the Presidio of San Francisco. GPS: N37 48.384' / W122 26.900'

(1) From the intersection of Market, Ninth, Hayes, and Larkin Streets near the Civic Center downtown, veer left onto Hayes and go 3 blocks. Turn right onto Franklin Street and go almost 2 miles to Bay Street. Turn left onto Bay and follow the traffic as it curves onto Laguna Street, and then onto Marina Boulevard. Continue on Marina Boulevard for 8 blocks to the stoplight just past the end of the West Harbor—where the Presidio's Mason Street meets Marina Boulevard and the Presidio Parkway. Go right at the light and drive 1 block along the edge of the grassy field to reach the shoreline parking lot immediately west of the St. Francis Yacht Club.

(2) From the Golden Gate Bridge, continue south on US 101 / Presidio Parkway to the Marina exit (stay in the left-hand lanes after you come off the bridge). Head left and take the next left onto Mason Street. The shoreline parking lot is just west of the St. Francis Yacht Club. Additional parking is available in the GGNRA parking lot between Mason Street and the shoreline, just west of where Mason meets Marina Boulevard.

Public transportation: San Francisco Municipal Railway (Muni) buses stop at the corner of Broderick and Jefferson Streets, 4 blocks from the start of this walk. Contact Muni for information about schedules, fares, and accessibility (sfmta.com, tripplanner.transit.511.org). The PresidioGo

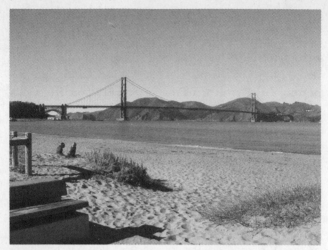
The beach bordering the Golden Gate Promenade offers a fabulous view of the namesake bridge.

Shuttle provides service within the Presidio of San Francisco, as well as routes that link downtown to the park. Visit presidiobus.com for maps and information.

Overview: A premier tour of the shoreline of San Francisco Bay, the Golden Gate Promenade rambles alongside a length of beach that was once a vast expanse of dune edged by salt marshes and lagoons, and later the site of a military landing strip and work yard. An astonishing feat of environmental restoration has revived the beachfront as a natural treasure; dubbed the Crissy Field Restoration Project, the combined efforts of the National Park Service's GGNRA, the Golden Gate National Parks Association (the GGNRA's nonprofit support partner), and several private foundations made the restoration possible.

Crissy Field, a military airstrip, was built in the 1920s, when flight was young. Constructed in peacetime and predating the US Air Force, the field housed the air squadron based at the Presidio and was used as a base for fire patrols and aerial-photography flights. In the restoration process the 100-acre field was cleared of all hazardous substances, the pavement removed, and the area replanted with grass. The neighboring beach was cleaned and widened, the promenade was surfaced in crushed stone, and a 20-acre tidal marsh was built, while the dunes that separate beach from marsh and field were planted with native species. The result: a length of shoreline that allows walkers to feel the sun on their faces or the bite of the fog, a beachfront that invites sunbathing and sand sports, an expanse of grass where dogs and children run free, a stunning visual palette, and links to a military legacy that dates back more than 200 years.

In addition to wandering along the shoreline, the Golden Gate Promenade leads past a historic Coast Guard station, out onto a public fishing pier, and to Fort Point, a Civil War–era brick fortification just beneath the southern anchor of the Golden Gate Bridge.

Note: The Golden Gate Promenade can be combined with the walk along the Marina Green (Walk 7) in a 7-mile leg-stretching ramble along the bay. The two walks meet in the parking lot just to the west of the St. Francis Yacht Club.

The Walk

▶The promenade formally begins at the edge of the parking lot on the west side of the St. Francis Yacht Club. But given that you may park in a different lot, taking any path toward the bay will land you on the broad, crushed-stone surface of the promenade. Head left (west), toward the

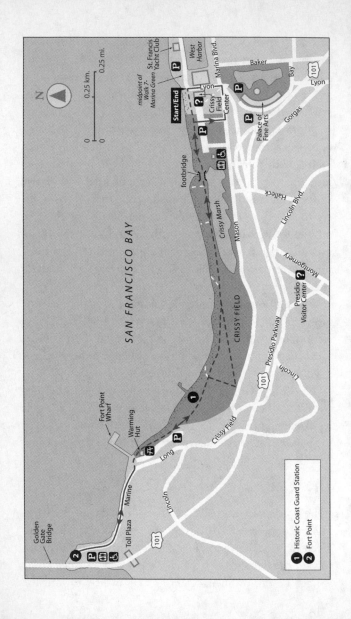

SAN FRANCISCO BAY

N

0.25 km.
0.25 mi.

Golden
Gate
Bridge

Toll Plaza

Marine

Fort Point
Wharf

Warming
Hut

Long

Crissy Field

Lincoln

Presidio Parkway

CRISSY FIELD

Crissy Marsh

Mason

footbridge

Start/End

Crissy
Field
Center

Lyon

midpoint of Walk 7-
Marina Green

St. Francis Yacht Club

West
Harbor

Marina Blvd.

Baker

Bay

Lyon

Gorgas

Palace of
Fine Arts

Halleck

Lincoln Blvd.

Montgomery

Presidio
Visitor Center

① Historic Coast Guard Station
② Fort Point

Golden Gate. Your immersion into a world of dunes, salt air, wind, and waves is immediate.

▶It's impossible to get lost on the promenade. A bank of dunes separates the walkway from the broad beach, and beach scrub, followed by the tidal marsh, borders on the inland side. The beach serves as a launch pad to one of the most popular windsurfing areas in the world. Stiff breezes and strong bay currents make the surfing here challenging; you're not likely to see novices in the waters. But experienced windsurfers make skimming across the bay at 25 to 30 knots (30 to 35 mph) look easy. For those not schooled in the sport, flying a kite is a much easier (and less hazardous) way to sample the wind.

▶Cross the footbridge that spans the inlet to the tidal marsh. The marsh is new, yet old. Originally marshland, this area was filled in and paved in the early part of the twentieth century to serve as part of Crissy Field. When the army turned the Presidio over to the National Park Service, the pavement of the airfield was removed and restoration began. Now the rebuilt marsh teems with birdlife, a happy return to a healthy habitat.

▶Pass the first of a number of paths that lead through the sand dunes to the beach. To preserve this carefully nurtured habitat, stay on the paths as you move between the promenade and the sand. Though a number of native plants survived on the dunes through years of abuse, the National Park Service planted more than 55,000 natives as part of the restoration. These included arrowgrass, rushes, pickleweed, salt grass, sea pink, and other members of the

FORT POINT

From the outside, Fort Point doesn't look like much. Blocky and plain, it resembles a brick warehouse, albeit one with a lighthouse and some narrow, odd-looking windows. The steel latticework supporting the Golden Gate Bridge, which was built over the site in the 1930s, holds more visual intrigue than the building in its shadow.

But on the inside the fort is an architectural marvel. Thick arches are mounted in three tiers, one atop the other, surrounding an open courtyard. Towers rise in three corners of the court, housing spiral staircases of thick granite that climb to the rooftop, which is open to the Golden Gate and views of San Francisco Bay and the San Francisco skyline.

The empty shadowy corridors on the west, north, and east sides of the fort, facing ocean and bay, are lined with alcoves, known as casements, that once housed Civil War–era cannons. The casements are now devoid of weaponry, their openings either bricked over or blocked with clouded glass. Living quarters—rooms with arched ceilings linked by a long corridor of open doors—line the south side of the fort on the second tier. Long emptied of the trappings of the officers that once resided there, the rooms now house interpretive displays describing the history of the fort.

The history of a defensive post at Fort Point dates back to the Spanish, who, with the help of local natives, erected a structure known as Castillo de San Joaquin in the early 1790s on the site. That fort was razed to make way for the present edifice, built between 1853 and 1861 by the US Army Corps of Engineers and first manned by a company of the Third US Artillery Regiment. The fort was designed to house 126 cannons, with casements for thirty guns on each tier, and was intended to defend San Francisco Bay from an invasion that never materialized.

The fort quickly became obsolete. By 1900 it was used for training, storage, and as an operational base during the construction of the Golden Gate Bridge in the 1930s. It was manned again during World War II, as part of the defensive network erected around the mouth of the bay, then again fell into disuse. Its current revival as a National Historic Site began in 1970, and today it is one of the most prominent attractions within the Golden Gate National Recreation Area.

Interpretative displays explaining the history and operation of the fort begin when you walk through the sally port. Be sure to climb to the barbette tier, on top of the fort. The perimeter is studded with massive gun emplacements, complete with the rusted metal fixtures used to mount the cannon. The stubby Fort Point Light stands on the westernmost border of the tier, the last of three lighthouses built on and around Fort Point in the 1850s and 1860s. The light was extinguished in 1934.

Fort Point is open Friday, Saturday, and Sunday from 10 a.m. to 5 p.m.; it is closed Monday through Thursday and on Thanksgiving, Christmas, and New Year's Day. You can take a tour led by a ranger or park volunteer, follow a self-guided tour, or rent a tour on tape. A printed interpretive guide of the fort is also available at the bookstore, as well as through the fort's website at nps.gov/fopo. For more information, call (415) 556-1693.

saltwater-marsh plant community, as well as plants from the coastal scrub plant community, which includes bush lupine, coyote brush, and monkeyflower. The plantings have a firm foothold but still don't deserve to be trampled. You can traverse between promenade and beach as often as you like, as a number of links foster easy passage between the two.

▶Leave the tidal marsh behind for the grassy expanse of Crissy Field. Paths weave across the elevated field. Continue west toward the Golden Gate, pausing to take in the views as whim dictates.

▶At the east end of the meadow, pick up a paved path that leads right, back down onto the promenade. Continue left on the waterside path, passing the historic Coast Guard station. The station's residence dates from 1890 and the boathouse from 1919. The Gulf of the Farallones National Marine Sanctuary visitor center occupies the station.

▶Continue on the promenade as it draws close to the water's edge. Pause to check in at the Warming Hut, which houses a cafe and gift shop. Restrooms are located in a separate, neighboring building. Just beyond, the Fort Point Wharf, built in 1908 and used today as a public fishing pier, juts out into the bay. On weekends the pier is often packed with sightseers and anglers.

▶The promenade ends on Marine Drive, which continues out to the Civil War–era Fort Point. Walk along the edge of Marine Drive toward the austere brick building, hulking in the shadows at the foot of the Golden Gate

CRISSY FIELD

Before Crissy Field began its incarnation as an airstrip, it had served the people of San Francisco and the soldiers of the Presidio in other ways. In the late 1800s it was used as a storage area and a dump—uses that seem unconscionable given its spectacular natural setting. In 1915 the tidal flats along the bay front were filled in preparation for the Panama-Pacific International Exposition. After the exposition the land was chosen by the army as a site for an Air Coast Defense Station, and the airfield was born.

In its early years aviators flew reconnaissance from Crissy Field and also took aerial photographs, went out on search-and-rescue missions, patrolled for forest fires, and even took part in dedication ceremonies for Lassen Volcanic National Park, which was dedicated in 1916 after the plug dome volcano blew its top in 1915.

By the mid-1930s, however, enthusiasm for Crissy Field as a "first-line air base" was waning. Fog and wind had always plagued the fliers (and is still responsible for delays at San Francisco International Airport). The completion of the Golden Gate Bridge in 1937, which compromised flight lines, sealed the airfield's demise. Crissy Field became part of the Golden Gate National Recreation Area when the Presidio was turned over to the National Park Service in 1994.

Bridge. Waves crash against the breakwater just to your right. Believe it or not, surfers can be found offshore here, catching rides toward a perilous shore.

▸Arrive at Fort Point and wander around the perimeter of the building for an intimate view of the colossal struts and anchor of the bridge, standing directly underneath its broad, clanging span. The water under the bridge churns with the powerful currents that roll through the Golden Gate. The mighty Pacific Ocean opens to the west.

▸When you're done checking out the exterior—and if the fort is open on the day of your visit—head through the sally port for an inside look (no fee is levied). Check out the main courtyard of the five-sided structure, then climb the stairs that lead to exhibits on the upper floors and then to the rooftop. There is no elevator access. The roof offers dramatic views of the bridge, the bay, the city, and the ocean and is unprotected from the seemingly perpetual wind funneled through the Golden Gate.

▸Exit Fort Point and return along the roadway to the shoreline promenade. Retrace your steps past the Coast Guard station, the grassy meadow, and the tidal marsh, following the promenade back to the parking lots near the St. Francis Yacht Club and the end of this walk.

PACIFIC COAST

Walk 9: Golden Gate Bridge and Baker Beach

General location: In northwestern San Francisco, south and west of the Golden Gate Bridge

Special attractions: Golden Gate Bridge; clifftop views of San Francisco, the Pacific Ocean, and San Francisco Bay; military landmarks; a broad expanse of beach

Difficulty: Moderate, with some steep climbs. The trail surface is narrow, uneven, and includes stretches of sand.

Distance: 4.0 miles

Estimated time: 2.5 hours

Services: Parking, restrooms, snack bar

Restrictions: Not wheelchair accessible. However, beach wheelchairs can be used on portions of the trail. Contact the Golden Gate National Recreation Area (GGNRA) at (415) 561-4700 a week in advance of your visit to reserve a chair. Be careful on cliffs and at the beaches. This part of the coastline is known for its strong riptides; Baker Beach is posted for hazardous surf. Each year the National Park Service rescues people who fall off cliffs or get swept away by heavy surf or riptides. Dogs must either be leashed or under voice control, depending on where you are walking in the GGNRA. In some areas pets are prohibited entirely to protect sensitive resources. Dog droppings must be picked up. Contact the GGNRA headquarters at Fort Mason for pet regulations. Note that improvements to the Batteries to Bluffs Trail were ongoing in 2013 and 2014; be prepared for realignments, especially between the Pacific Overlook and Battery Godfrey.

For more information: Golden Gate National Recreation Area, Fort Mason, Building 201, San Francisco, CA 94123-0022; (415) 561-4700; nps.gov/goga

Getting started: This walk begins at the entrance to Battery Chamberlin at Baker Beach. GPS: N37 47.589' / W122 28.996'

(1) From the intersection of Market, Ninth, Hayes, and Larkin Streets, veer left onto Hayes and go 3 blocks. Turn right onto Franklin Street and go about 1.75 miles to Lombard Street. Turn left onto Lombard to its end, curving right with traffic onto Park Presidio and the approach to the Golden Gate Bridge. Follow Park Presidio for a little more than 1 mile to the last exit before the toll plaza on the bridge. Go right on the exit and circle around to the stop sign. Turn right onto Lincoln Boulevard and follow it for about 1 mile to Bowley Street. Make a right turn onto Bowley and proceed 0.2 mile to Gibson Road. Follow Gibson Road for about 1 block, then make a right turn onto Battery Chamberlin Road. Park in the lot at the end of Battery Chamberlin Road, which runs alongside Baker Beach. The trail begins at the far end of the lot, by the fence surrounding the battery.

(2) From the San Francisco Peninsula, follow I-280 north through Daly City. Take the Golden Gate Bridge / 19th Avenue exit (stay in left-hand lanes on the freeway) and follow CA 1 north—along Junipero Serra Boulevard and 19th Avenue—for about 5 miles. Stay in

the left lane as you enter Golden Gate Park, and go left at the light onto Crossover Drive. At Fulton Street continue straight on 25th Avenue. Follow 25th Avenue for 1 mile to El Camino del Mar. Go right on El Camino del Mar, which merges onto Lincoln Boulevard, for about 0.5 mile, then turn left onto Bowley Street. Follow Bowley to Gibson, Gibson to Battery Chamberlin, and Battery Chamberlin to the parking lot at the trailhead.

(3) From the southbound lanes of US 101 at the Golden Gate Bridge, pass through the far right tollbooth, take an immediate right at the 25th Avenue exit, and continue onto Merchant Road. From Merchant Road turn left at the first stop sign onto Lincoln Boulevard. Follow Lincoln Boulevard for about 1 mile to Bowley Street. Follow Bowley to Gibson, Gibson to Battery Chamberlin, and Battery Chamberlin to the parking lot at the trailhead.

Public transportation: San Francisco Municipal Railway (Muni) buses stop near the junction of Bowley Street and Lincoln Boulevard. Contact Muni for information about schedules, fares, and accessibility (sfmta.com, tripplanner .transit.511.org). The PresidioGo Shuttle provides service within the Presidio of San Francisco, as well as routes that link downtown to the park. Visit presidiobus.com for maps and information.

Overview: While there's no denying that the main draw of this walk/hike is the Golden Gate Bridge, a loop along the bluffs between Baker Beach and the bridge itself brims with beautiful vistas and provocative historic sites. The Golden Gate is a tangible symbol of the vitality, elegance, and strength of the City by the Bay; the wall-to-wall batteries on the headlands flanking the spectacular structure

GOLDEN GATE BRIDGE

Perhaps the most photogenic—and photographed—bridge in the world, the Golden Gate Bridge is vivid and compelling. A lifetime of driving over the span never dulls the thrill: The towers draw your eye up to the heavens, and there isn't a San Franciscan on the planet who doesn't gaze westward as they cross, to see if the Farallon Islands are visible. If they are, there's a good chance the fog won't roll in.

Built by engineer Joseph Strauss and designed by architect Irving Morrow, the bridge took more than four years to construct, from 1933 to 1937. The cost was $35 million. The 6,450-foot span was the longest in the world at the time of its completion, and the cable that suspends the span would stretch 80,000

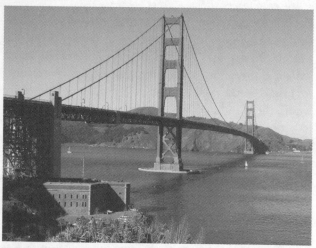

Fort Point hunkers beneath the southern anchorage of the Golden Gate Bridge.

miles, or about three times around the earth, were it to come unspun.

This feat of engineering and artistry carries more than 100,000 vehicles to and from the city each day. Pedestrians often crowd the walkway on the bridge's east side, while the walkway on the west is reserved for bicyclists.

If you want to walk across the bridge—about 1.7 miles each way—set out from the bridge's Strauss Plaza. It's a quintessential San Francisco experience but one that you'll likely only choose to enjoy once. The walk is enervating in a number of ways, including its proximity to traffic, the abrupt drop to the bay or the Pacific (220 feet from the span to mean high water), and the incessant wind and fog funneling through the gate. But it's a bucket-list achievement, even for locals. Just keep in mind that viewing the bridge from a distance can be just as rewarding as feeling it vibrate under your feet.

For more information about the bridge—everything from a photo gallery and bridge statistics to ways to pay tolls—visit goldengatebridge.org.

symbolize just how hard its residents—and a nation—were prepared to fight to protect it.

The walk begins at Baker Beach, with passage through Battery Chamberlin. A restored "disappearing" gun is mounted in the first emplacement at the old battery. This weapon was designed to drop out of sight after discharging so that artillerymen could reload it. If you visit on the first weekend of the month, a park ranger and volunteers in period uniform will be on hand to describe how the gun operated.

Beyond the battery the sandy path leads up and alongside busy Lincoln Boulevard, with views spreading north across the channel to the Marin Headlands. It's a bit of a climb, but the Golden Gate Bridge will spur you on. Closer to the bridge a series of batteries constructed over nearly one hundred years, from the Civil War to World War II, line the route. The batteries are poignant to explore—where once there were weapons, now there are photographers, tourists, and walkers who use the concrete aprons to visit, read, picnic, and sunbathe.

The stunning architecture of the bridge is the exclamation point near the turnaround of this walk. The route dives under the span, and the architecture, surprisingly lacy, arcs overhead. Check out the exhibits in the bridge plaza before returning down battery row.

Where the batteries appear to end, nature takes over. A slender path composed of staircases and dirt drops to a tiny beach with enormous views. From there the trail climbs through the native scrub—vibrant California poppies, feathery yarrow, brittle ceanothus—to Battery Crosby, tucked into the scrub. Take the Sand Ladder down to Baker Beach and end your journey on the sand, surrounded by other beachgoers and treated to more great views—these of the posh homes of Seacliff and the dark walls of Lands End.

Note: The easternmost reaches of Baker Beach are clothing-optional. Stick to the high ground if you'd like to avoid this part of the shoreline.

The Walk

►Start by walking through the beach-side opening in the chain-link fence at Battery Chamberlin. Walk up and along the concrete aprons fronting the four gun emplacements, then bear right and up on the obvious Coastal Trail.

►The broad, obvious path leads up through the woods to the side of Lincoln Boulevard at 0.5 mile. Go left, following the roadside path uphill and enjoying the amazing views (if the fog permits) out across the channel to the Marin Headlands.

►Pass the signed trail on the left for the Sand Ladder. You'll take that down to the beach on the downhill run.

►Pass the signed trail to Battery Crosby, staying right on the path that runs alongside Lincoln Boulevard. You will use this path on the return trip as well.

►Pause at the Pacific Overlook (1 mile). The benches and the views invite you to sit and stay a while, watching the maritime traffic move through the Golden Gate.

►Reach the top of the climb, where the Coastal Trail turns left, heading into a stand of trees and away from Lincoln Boulevard. Follow the signed Batteries to Bluffs Trail toward the water and the Golden Gate Bridge.

►Stay right at the fork in the woods, heading toward the bridge.

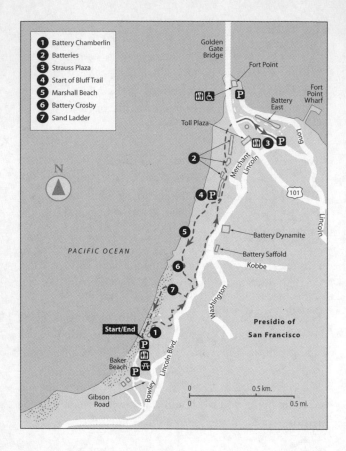

1 Battery Chamberlin
2 Batteries
3 Strauss Plaza
4 Start of Bluff Trail
5 Marshall Beach
6 Battery Crosby
7 Sand Ladder

Golden Gate Bridge

Fort Point

Fort Point Wharf

Battery East

Toll Plaza

Long

Merchant

Lincoln

101

Lincoln

PACIFIC OCEAN

Battery Dynamite

Battery Saffold

Kobbe

Washington

Presidio of San Francisco

Start/End

Baker Beach

Lincoln Blvd

Bowley

Gibson Road

0   0.5 km.

0   0.5 mi.

▶Reach Battery Godfrey, the first concrete installation along the trail. The wide concrete apron atop the battery faces the Golden Gate and makes a marvelous bench from which to enjoy the views. Battery Godfrey melds into Battery Boutelle at 1.2 miles. You can explore the batteries at will, but the main route stays to the right, dropping down a flight of steps and passing Battery Marcus Miller and Battery Cranston.

▸At the base of the staircase, the route broadens, becomes paved, and drops toward the Golden Gate Bridge, which now dominates everything about the trail. A yellow line splits traffic on the heavily used path, and you'll need to be aware of cyclists using the route to access or leave the bridge. Stay on the path; ongoing restoration efforts seek to reestablish native habitat at the bridge approach, including such rare plant species as coast rock cress and San Francisco gum plant. Serpentine habitats, underlain by serpentinite, the state rock of California, once stretched in a band across the San Francisco Peninsula.

▸Follow the pavement to the left (north, then east), dropping under the roadbed of the bridge. The sound of the cars passing overhead is hollow, muffled, and echoing; the architecture is intricate, solid, and insulating. Watch for speeding cyclists. An interpretive site on the west side of the span includes a re-creation of the metalwork that supports the bridge at the southern and northern anchorages.

▸As you emerge from the shadow of the bridge on the east side of the Golden Gate, Fort Point comes into view below and to the left (north). Carefully cross the busy pathway, heading right and slightly uphill toward the bridge's Strauss Plaza (2 miles). The plaza is busy and inviting, with a kaleidoscopic diorama that shows the various stages of the bridge's construction, a statue of bridge builder Joseph Strauss, and exhibits that document the bridge's construction. The plaza is also home to the Roundhouse Gift Center and Bridge Cafe, public restrooms, and the beginning of the pedestrian walkway across the Golden Gate Bridge. In addition, you can follow paths that lead down past

COASTAL GUN EMPLACEMENTS

Defensive fortifications at the Golden Gate date back to the Spanish occupation, when the Castillo de San Joaquin was established on the site where Fort Point now stands. Fort Point, along with a fort on Alcatraz Island, was armed in 1861, with the purpose of protecting the entrance to San Francisco Bay from enemies intent on stealing the wealth of the city after the discovery of gold in 1848, and from the rebels during the Civil War.

Improvements in weaponry eventually rendered these huge brick forts obsolete, and new fortifications, able to withstand new technologies, were built into the headlands at Batteries West and East in the 1870s. Earthworks, now covered in grasses and flowers, protected the guns sheltered in these batteries—and the men who manned them—from enemy ordnance. But by the late 1800s, the earthwork batteries had also become dangerously passé. Under the direction of two secretaries of war, William Endicott and William Taft, the Presidio broke out in new batteries like it had the chicken pox. Over a period of about twenty years, the Presidio (actually, technically, Fort Winfield Scott, which was later incorporated into the Presidio) gained Batteries Chamberlin, Crosby, Stotsenburg-McKinnon, Stafford, Dynamite, Godfrey, Boutelle, Marcus Miller, Cranston, Howe-Wagner, Lancaster, Baldwin, Sherwood, Slaughter, and Blaney. These batteries feature a predictable but vaguely individual architecture and purpose. Case in point: the disappearing gun

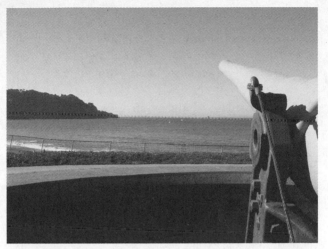

Battery Chamberlin's disappearing gun takes aim at Lands End.

at Battery Chamberlin. Another example: Battery Dynamite, which was outfitted with guns that fired charges of dynamite that proved useless for combat but, according to a park report on the history of seacoast fortifications, "killed prodigious numbers of fish when test fired."

For all that was invested over the years in military fortifications around the Golden Gate, there was never a need to use them. A shot was never fired on an enemy from any of the batteries at the Presidio. Some might assert that the apparent strength of these fortifications deterred potential attackers, but then again, San Francisco may have just been lucky.

Battery East to Crissy Field, Fort Point, and the Golden Gate Promenade. (**Note**: The Roundhouse and Bridge Cafe were undergoing renovation starting in 2014. Visit goldengatebridge.org/gift for more information.)

▶When you are ready, retrace your steps under the bridge and past the row of batteries. At the end of the battery row, before the trail bends left to parallel Lincoln Boulevard, stay right on the dirt path. Pass brickwork openings in the bluff to the left, which are part of Battery West, which dates from the post–Civil War era.

▶The dirt path ends at a T junction. Go right on the signed Bluffs Trail, which drops steeply down the scrub-covered hillside via a well-built stairway.

▶Pass a viewpoint on the right. The peaceful path is punctuated by flights of wooden stairs.

▶Arrive at the base of the bluffs and Marshall Beach (3.3 miles). The little beach opens onto a big ocean, with staggering views of the Golden Gate and the Marin Headlands.

▶Begin the climb up to Battery Crosby. The route is broken up with staircases; check out the rocks in the trail, which are serpentine and soapstone worn shiny by the passage of many feet.

▶The climb deposits you in front of the gun emplacements of Battery Crosby, which offer yet another great viewpoint. Follow the relatively flat path back to the Coastal Trail parallel to Lincoln Boulevard.

▶Turn right, walk about 0.1 mile down the Coastal Trail, then turn right on the signed Sand Ladder trail. Steep and sandy, lined by cables and featuring log steps, the ladder is no joke: It pretty much drops you straight down onto Baker Beach.

▶Turn left once you reach the beach, and walk through the sand back toward Battery Chamberlin and the parking area, both of which are in sight. You can either take the stair-step path that leads up to the battery or continue down the beach to the parking lot, which is open to the beach.

Walk 10: Ocean Beach

♿ 🌿 👪 ✕ 📷

General location: In northwestern San Francisco, on the western edge of Golden Gate Park and along the Pacific Ocean

Special attractions: Beach walking; sea lion and shorebird viewing; historic architecture and murals; a formal garden

Difficulty: Easy

Distance: 1.9 miles

Estimated time: 1 hour

Services: Parking, restaurants, restrooms

Restrictions: Wheelchair accessible only along the Ocean Beach Esplanade. Beach wheelchairs can be used on portions of the route. Contact the GGNRA at (415) 561-4700 a week in advance of your visit to reserve a chair. The hill up to the Cliff House is rather steep but may be accessible to wheelchairs. Dogs must be leashed and their droppings picked up. On Ocean Beach dogs are allowed if kept under voice control from Sloat Boulevard north to Stairwell 21, where leashes are required all year to protect the endangered snowy plover, except from May 15 to July 1. Be careful on cliffs and at the beach. Each year the park service rescues numerous people who fall off cliffs or get swept away by heavy surf or riptides.

For more information: Golden Gate National Recreation Area, Fort Mason, Building 201, San Francisco, CA 94123-0022; (415) 561-4700; nps.gov/goga

Getting started: This walk starts at the Dutch Windmill and Queen Wilhelmina Tulip Garden. GPS: N37 46.204' / W122 30.555'

(1) From the intersection of Market, Ninth, Hayes, and Larkin Streets near the Civic Center, veer left onto Hayes and go 3 blocks. Turn right onto Franklin Street and go 9 blocks. Turn left onto Geary Boulevard and drive approximately 5 miles to the Pacific Ocean. About 0.5 mile before you reach the shoreline, veer right with traffic onto Point Lobos Avenue and follow Point Lobos to the coast. Once at ocean level continue on the Great Highway for about 0.5 mile to the Beach Chalet, 1.5 blocks beyond Fulton Street.

(2) From the San Francisco Peninsula, follow I-280. After passing through Daly City, take the Golden Gate Bridge/19th Avenue exit (stay in the left lanes of the freeway), and follow CA 1 north, along Junipero Serra Boulevard, 19th Avenue, and Park Presidio Boulevard, for about 4 miles to Irving Street. Turn right onto Irving and go 1 block. Turn left onto 18th Avenue and go 1 block. Turn left onto Lincoln Way and drive 2 miles to the Pacific Ocean. Turn right onto the Great Highway and drive about half a mile to the Beach Chalet.

(3) From the Golden Gate Bridge southbound, pass through the far right tollbooth, take an immediate right at the 25th Avenue exit, and continue onto Merchant Road. At the first stop sign, turn right onto Lincoln Boulevard and drive on Lincoln for about 1.5 miles. Just after Lincoln emerges from the Presidio, turn left onto 25th Avenue and go 4 blocks. Turn right onto Geary Boulevard and drive approximately 1.5 miles to the Pacific Ocean. In the last 0.5 mile, veer right with the traffic onto Point Lobos Avenue. Continue on Point Lobos to the coast. Once at ocean level continue on the Great Highway for about 0.5 mile to the Beach Chalet, 1.5 blocks beyond Fulton Street.

You might be able to find parking in the Beach Chalet lot, but it's more likely you'll end up alongside John F. Kennedy Drive in Golden Gate Park or in the linear parking lot between the Great Highway and the ocean.

Public transportation: San Francisco Municipal Railway (Muni) buses run from downtown to the end of Fulton at the Great Highway, about a half block from the Dutch Windmill and from the Beach Chalet. Buses also run to the junction of Judah and the Great Highway, roughly 4 blocks south of the Beach Chalet. Contact Muni for information about schedules, fares, and accessibility (sfmta .com, tripplanner.transit.511.org).

Overview: Most of the time Ocean Beach is shrouded in fog. With nothing to the west but the open ocean, nothing overhead but thick, flat grayness, gliding sea gulls, and perhaps the faint white orb of the sun as it sinks toward the western horizon, and nothing to be heard over the crashing surf, everything else that is San Francisco, beginning just on the other side of the seawall, might be forgotten.

Then again, particularly on sunny days, Ocean Beach pops with activity. Games of ultimate Frisbee and tag football, kites whirling overhead, sailboarders and surfers catching waves, and, of course, people walking the esplanade mingle with sunbathers and sand castle builders. The famous Cliff House rides above it all, classy and romantic on its end-of-the-continent perch.

The stroll—this is definitely not a vigorous hike—begins in Golden Gate Park, with a visit to a Dutch windmill and tulip garden. You then cross the Great Highway to walk along one of San Francisco's finest public beaches. You can walk on the sand or on the paved esplanade just above, using any of the short staircases to either access the beach

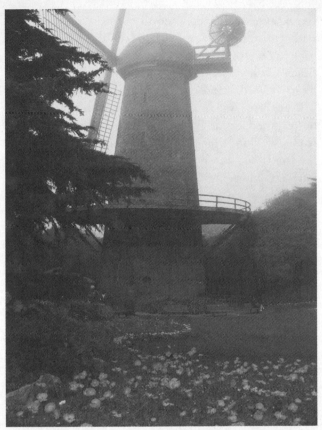
Fog shrouds the Dutch Windmill on the western border of Golden Gate Park.

or leave it. Follow the esplanade up to the Cliff House, all dolled up in shiny glass and whitewashed curves. Here you can savor a cocktail, indulge in a glorious meal with a glorious view, visit the gift shop, or simply walk around the patios that circle the historic site. Look south down the expanse of the beach, north onto the ruins of Sutro Baths, or west past Seal Rocks to the Pacific. When you have had your fill, stroll back down the beach to visit the Beach Chalet, checking out its panoramic murals before returning to the city's clamor.

Note: This walk may be combined with a longer journey on the Coastal Trail at Lands End. Linking the two requires walking a long block along Point Lobos Avenue to the Lands End Visitor Center in the Merrie Way parking lot. The walk along Lands End begins on the north side of the lot.

The Walk

▶Start at the towering Dutch Windmill on John F. Kennedy Drive, which was built in 1903 to pump water from freshwater wells to irrigate Golden Gate Park and, in the words of the Park Commission, to "lend to the landscape a picturesque feature." A second windmill, the Murphy Windmill, located on the south side of the linear park, was built at the same time. Both windmills were obsolete by 1913, as wind power was replaced by motorized pumps. The Dutch Windmill was restored in 1981; the Murphy Windmill was restored and reopened in 2012.

▶Explore the Queen Wilhelmina Tulip Garden adjacent to the windmill. Whatever the season and even on the foggiest San Francisco morning, this garden sparkles with bright colors laid out in orderly patterns. In early spring (February or March), you will find a dazzling display of tulips, as many as 10,000 of them. A host of other flowering plants bloom here during the remainder of the year.

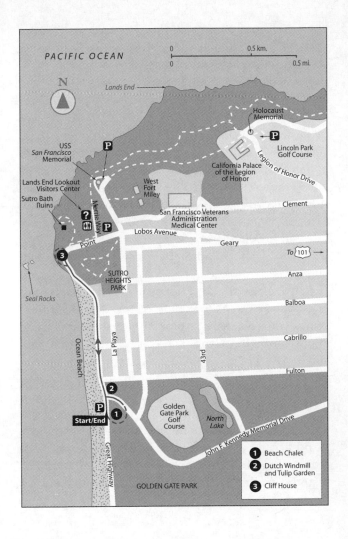

PACIFIC OCEAN

0   0.5 km.

0   0.5 mi.

N

Lands End

USS *San Francisco* Memorial

Lands End Lookout Visitors Center

Sutro Bath Ruins

Seal Rocks

Nettie Way

Point

SUTRO HEIGHTS PARK

Ocean Beach

La Playa

Start/End

Great Highway

GOLDEN GATE PARK

West Fort Miley

San Francisco Veterans Administration Medical Center

Lobos Avenue

Geary

Anza

Balboa

Cabrillo

Fulton

43rd

Golden Gate Park Golf Course

North Lake

John F. Kennedy Memorial Drive

Holocaust Memorial

Lincoln Park Golf Course

California Palace of the Legion of Honor

Legion of Honor Drive

Clement

To 101

1 Beach Chalet

2 Dutch Windmill and Tulip Garden

3 Cliff House

THE CLIFF HOUSE

The story goes that California sea lions and harbor seals, which gather to sun and swim at Seal Rocks, and have entertained sightseers since the middle of the nineteenth century, initially inspired a New York investor to build a resort at the site of what is now the Cliff House in 1863. That first Cliff House was relatively low-key, especially when compared to its successor, but still drew some of the finest families in San Francisco, as well as three presidents, to its dining rooms. Purchased by San Francisco millionaire Adolph Sutro in 1881 as part of his acquisition of a number of holdings at Point Lobos, the first structure was heavily damaged when a schooner carrying dynamite ran aground on the rocks below the building and exploded.

Sutro rebuilt the Cliff House in grand style: Haunting pictures of this iteration of the Cliff House are printed on postcards and posters that can be found in gift shops throughout the city. Sutro's spectacular, turreted, Gothic-style structure stood on the site for little more than ten years before it, too, was destroyed by fire. The third Cliff House, more modest than Sutro's, was opened in 1909 by his daughter, Emma, and was renovated several times before being acquired by the Golden Gate National Recreation Area in 1977. The most recent remodel has restored the neoclassical facade of Emma Sutro's vision.

▶Return to the Great Highway, turn right, and walk a partial block to Fulton Street. Cross the Great Highway with the light at Fulton.

▶Turn right and walk along the esplanade toward the Cliff House. To walk at the water's edge, descend to the sand at one of the many stairways cut into the concrete retaining wall along the esplanade. Although you may see people in the water, Ocean Beach is known for its riptides, and swimming can be extremely dangerous.

▶The esplanade steepens as it approaches the Cliff House, restored to its 1909 neoclassical appearance. Turn left off the main sidewalk before you reach the main entrance and follow the walkway that circles behind the building. You can look down, over the wall, at dizzying views of breakers hitting the rocks below, and back southward at the great stretch of Ocean Beach. From this vantage point you can see both windmills in Golden Gate Park. The modern apartment complex that occupies the east side of the Great Highway just south of the Cliff House stands on the site of Playland at the Beach, an amusement park that delighted generations of San Franciscans. Playland closed in 1972.

▶Continue on the walkway to the oceanside patio behind the Cliff House. Look out over the ocean, and listen for the barking of the California sea lions that congregate on Seal Rocks, just offshore. You may also see a fishing boat heading out to sea or a freighter on the horizon. The ruins of the historic Sutro Baths can be seen from the north side of the patio.

The giant Camera Obscura and Holograph Gallery, a last remnant of Playland at the Beach, also still resides on the Cliff House patio. Claimed to be the world's biggest camera, the rotating San Francisco Camera Obscura captures haunting images of its surroundings—the plaza, the Seal Rocks, sunsets—on a large parabolic screen.

▸Retrace your steps across the patio and rejoin the esplanade, which passes in front of the Cliff House. You may want to step inside the Cliff House for a drink, a meal, or a visit to the gift shop. Visit cliffhouse.com for menus, hours, and information about present-day offerings in this historic structure.

▸Leaving the Cliff House, walk down the esplanade to Ocean Beach. Follow the esplanade or wander the beach back to the crosswalk at Fulton. Retrace your steps back to John F. Kennedy Drive, then cross to the south side, walk half a block, and reach the Beach Chalet. Built in 1925 to house a restaurant and changing rooms for Ocean Beach bathers, the Beach Chalet was designed by architect Willis Polk in the Spanish Colonial style and decorated in the late 1930s by muralist Lucien Labaudt. Labaudt's colorful scenes of San Francisco—commissioned by the Works Progress Administration—survive today. The chalet itself, renovated in 1996, is once again home to a restaurant and microbrewery.

▸To finish the walk, exit the Beach Chalet and return to wherever it was you found parking.

Walk 11: Lands End

🍴 🌿 👫 📷

General location: This walk skirts the bluffs along the Pacific coast outside the Golden Gate in northwestern San Francisco, just north of Ocean Beach and the Cliff House.

Special attractions: Natural landscapes; ocean, bridge, and city views; a museum; historic monuments; visitor center and cafe

Difficulty: Moderate, following dirt paths and including steep flights of stairs

Distance: 5.0 miles

Estimated time: 3 hours

Services: Restaurants, restrooms, parking, visitor information center

Restrictions: Not wheelchair accessible. Be careful on the cliffs and if you visit the beach. Each year the National Park Service rescues numerous people who fall off cliffs or get swept away by heavy surf or riptides. Dogs must be leashed, and droppings must be picked up. Contact the Golden Gate National Recreation Area (GGNRA) for the most current pet regulations.

For more information: Golden Gate National Recreation Area, Fort Mason, Building 201, San Francisco, CA 94123-0022; (415) 561-4700; nps.gov/goga. The Lands End visitor center, called Lands End Lookout, is at 680 Point Lobos Ave.; (415) 426-5240. The California Palace of the Legion of Honor in Lincoln Park is at 100 34th Ave.; (415) 750-3600; legionofhonor.famsf.org.

Getting started: This walk begins at the large parking lot on Merrie Way, off Point Lobos Avenue just above the Cliff House. GPS: N37 46.797' / W122 30.709'

(1) From the intersection of Market, Ninth, Hayes, and Larkin Streets near the Civic Center, veer left onto Hayes and go 3 blocks. Turn right onto Franklin Street and go 9 blocks. Turn left onto Geary Boulevard and drive approximately 5 miles to the Pacific Ocean. In the last 0.5 mile, veer right, with traffic, onto Point Lobos Avenue. Continue on Point Lobos for 0.75 mile, turn right on Merrie Way, and park in the lot.

(2) From the San Francisco Peninsula, follow I-280 northbound. After passing through Daly City, take the Golden Gate Bridge / 19th Avenue exit (stay in the left-hand lanes of the freeway), and drive on CA 1 north—along Junipero Serra Boulevard, 19th Avenue, and Park Presidio Boulevard—for about 4 miles to Irving Street. Turn right onto Irving and go 1 block. Turn left onto 18th Avenue and go 1 block. Turn left onto Lincoln Way and drive 2 miles to the Pacific Ocean. Turn right onto the Great Highway and drive about 1 mile. Follow traffic onto Point Lobos Avenue, winding up past the Cliff House. About 1 block past the Cliff House, turn left onto Merrie Way and park in the lot.

(3) From the southbound lanes of the Golden Gate Bridge (US 101), pass through the far right tollbooth, take an immediate right on the 25th Avenue exit, and continue onto Merchant Road. Turn right at the first stop sign onto Lincoln Boulevard. Drive on Lincoln for about 1.5 miles. Turn left onto 25th Avenue just after Lincoln emerges from the Presidio, and go 4 blocks. Turn right onto Geary Boulevard and drive approximately 1.5 miles toward the

Pacific Ocean. In the last 0.5 mile, veer right with the traffic onto Point Lobos Avenue. Continue on Point Lobos for 0.75 mile, turn right onto Merrie Way, and park in the lot.

Public transportation: San Francisco Municipal Railway (Muni) buses run from downtown to the Merrie Way junction on Point Lobos Avenue. Contact Muni for information about schedules, fares, and accessibility (sfmta .com, tripplanner.transit.511.org).

Overview: On a clear day this walk is sensational. Views from the Coastal Trail open across the Pacific all the way to the Farallon Islands and beyond, across the strait to the Marin Headlands and north to Point Reyes, and east to the Golden Gate Bridge. The loop also encompasses a magnificent museum, a chance to walk a labyrinth, a tour of the ruins of the historic Sutro Baths, and one of San Francisco's best-kept secrets, Sutro Heights Park. It's not an easy route, with several long staircases leading to and from the sights, but adding a workout to a walk is not a bad thing.

Beginning just uphill from the fabled Cliff House and the ruins of the Sutro Baths, the walk begins on the Coastal Trail. This clearly defined pathway, paved to start and becoming gravel as it rounds Point Lobos, provides both broad vistas and intimate glimpses of passing freighters, the remnants of shipwrecks at low tide, and the open ocean as it is funneled through the Golden Gate into San Francisco Bay. Because the cliffs can be unstable, stay on the trail at all times and keep a close eye on children in your party.

Midway through the walk you will emerge from the coastal forest into Lincoln Park, where golf carts and caddies wend across groomed greens. The California Palace of the Legion of Honor, one of San Francisco's fine city museums, is surrounded by the links. Upon leaving the Palace, reenter the forest and head back toward the point via a trail higher up the bluffs than the Coastal Trail but just as beautiful. At the end of the path, you will reach the moving memorial to the World War II heroics of the USS *San Francisco*.

Drop down through the Merrie Way parking lot to pick up the staircase that leads down to the ruins of Sutro Baths, a seaside draw for thousands of San Franciscans in the early twentieth century. Near the walk's end, climb gently up into Sutro Heights Park. This sanctuary, with its palm trees, spectacular views, and soothing open spaces, was the site of millionaire Adolph Sutro's extravagant country mansion and sculpture garden.

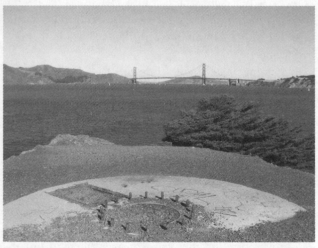

The studs of a gun emplacement punctuate an overlook of the Golden Gate Bridge at Lands End.

Be sure to start or end your walk with a tour of the GGNRA's Lands End visitor center, which offers interpretive materials, information, gifts, a cafe, restrooms, and water.

Note: If you hanker for some beach walking, you can add a stroll along Ocean Beach (Walk 10) to the beginning or end of the Lands End walk. To link the walks, from the Merrie Way parking lot, head downhill 1 long block to the Cliff House, and then continue down Ocean Beach to the Dutch Windmill and the Beach Chalet.

The Walk

▶Start at the trailhead at the far end of the Merrie Way parking lot, marked by a sign for the Coastal Trail.

▶Walk along the wide, paved (often sand-covered) path bordered by flowering shrubs and wildflowers. The green-blue ocean glitters through the Monterey pines, and you are likely to hear sea lions barking. The broad trail winds around the headland, curling eastward, with views opening across the strait of the Golden Gate.

▶Stop at the overlook at 0.3 mile, from which you can see a buoy shaped like a giant soda can. This buoy marks Mile Rock and warns inbound ships of the hazard. Across the channel you can see the Point Bonita Lighthouse, also designed to help ships safely enter the largest harbor on the West Coast. A staircase leads up to Fort Miley; stay straight on the broad Coastal Trail.

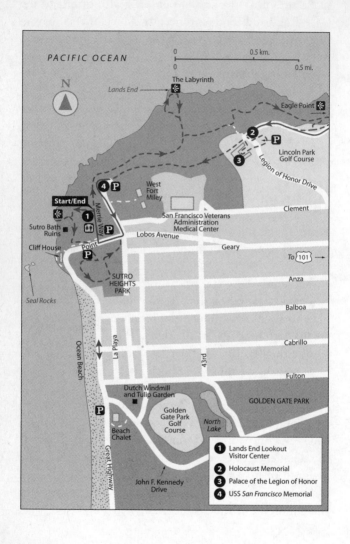

PACIFIC OCEAN

| 0 | | 0.5 km. |
| 0 | | 0.5 mi. |

N

Lands End

The Labyrinth

Eagle Point

Lincoln Park
Golf Course

2 Holocaust Memorial

3 Palace of the Legion of Honor

Legion of Honor Drive

4 USS San Francisco Memorial

West
Fort
Miley

Start/End

1 Lands End Lookout Visitor Center

Clement

Sutro Bath
Ruins

San Francisco Veterans
Administration
Medical Center

Lobos Avenue

Merrie Way

Cliff House

Point

Geary

To 101 →

Anza

SUTRO
HEIGHTS
PARK

Seal Rocks

Balboa

La Playa

43rd

Cabrillo

Ocean Beach

Fulton

Dutch Windmill
and Tulip Garden

GOLDEN GATE PARK

Golden
Gate Park
Golf
Course

North
Lake

Beach
Chalet

Great Highway

John F. Kennedy
Drive

1 Lands End Lookout
Visitor Center

2 Holocaust Memorial

3 Palace of the Legion of Honor

4 USS San Francisco Memorial

▶Another viewpoint offers more views of the Mile Rock buoy and across the channel onto the Marin Headlands. Pass the staircase that leads up to the Veterans Administration Hospital, then turn left and start down the steep staircase leading to the labyrinth.

▶At the base of the first flight of stairs, stay right on a narrow dirt path that leads out onto a point. A pair of gun emplacements dating back to the battery days flank a labyrinth constructed of ocean-smoothed stones. Take the time to walk the labyrinth: Your meditation will be bathed in sea breezes and accompanied by the sounding of the buoy.

▶From the labyrinth, follow the path to the west down to the little beach below.

▶A staircase climbs from the beach back to the "landing" where the path to the labyrinth begins. Stay right, climbing the stairs back to the Coastal Trail. Resume the walk by turning left.

▶At Painted Rock Cliff (1.5 miles), ascend a staircase built of railroad ties. A couple of rock benches on the long, long climb offer rest for weary legs and lungs.

▶At the top of the stairs, continue on the sandy path through a shady eucalyptus grove. Crescent-shaped eucalyptus leaves litter the forest floor. The route curves northward, toward the water, and descends a flight of easy stairs to an overlook.

▸The Coastal Trail parallels the Lincoln Park Golf Course to the overlook at Eagle Point, and ends just beyond, on the sidewalk next to El Camino del Mar. Turn right and follow the asphalt path alongside the golf course back uphill toward the California Palace of the Legion of Honor. Watch for golf cart traffic.

▸Use crosswalks near the apex of the climb to turn left toward the Palace of the Legion of Honor. Walk across Legion of Honor Drive to the sculpture created by American artist George Segal in memory of the victims of the Nazi Holocaust. This moving memorial—often strewn with flowers—is just downslope from the left (north) edge of the large parking lot in front of the museum.

▸Walk around the perimeter of the parking lot. Note the elegant period lampposts along the semicircular promenade, in keeping with the neoclassical museum—reminiscent of the Palais de la Legion d'Honneur in Paris. This beautifully designed overlook offers great city views, including, from left to right, the Transamerica Pyramid; the bold, dark Bank of America building; the University of San Francisco campus; and the University of California–San Francisco Medical Center at the base of Mount Parnassus.

▸Walk up the promenade to the entrance of the museum, past the formal garden. The statue in the center of the colonnade is a cast of French sculptor Auguste Rodin's *The Thinker*, its toe rubbed shiny by many an admiring schoolchild. Inside the palace is one of the world's most extensive collections of Rodin's sculptures. Aside from the Rodins, the museum houses collections representing the art of ancient Egypt and Rome; European painting, sculpture, and decorative arts from medieval times to the mid-twentieth century; and works of graphic arts. The museum's Achenbach Foundation for Graphic Arts collection includes more than 70,000 prints, drawings, and illustrated books, making it one of the largest of its kind in the United States.

▶Upon leaving the museum (2.5 miles), take an immediate left and walk down a gravel path to a set of concrete stairs. Descend the stairs, cross the driveway that runs beside the museum, and take a left into the parking lot just beyond.

▶Descend to the end of the parking lot (2.9 miles), pass through the gate, and pick up the dirt path marked with a GGNRA sign for the Coastal Trail and El Camino Del Mar. Walk down a railroad-tie stairway leading off to the right.

▶The path curves through a shady glen and through what, at some times of the year, is a forest of head-high wild fennel. Other paths lead downhill from the main path; stay on the level main trail.

▶Emerge from the coastal woods at the edge of the broad oval parking lot serving Fort Miley (3.3 miles), and walk along its perimeter for a sweeping view of the ocean, the Marin Headlands, and on a clear day, the Point Reyes peninsula far to the north. At the western edge of the lot, you will find a memorial to the USS *San Francisco* and the men who died on the cruiser in the Battle of Guadalcanal in

November 1942. Made from the battle-scarred bridge of the ship, the memorial bears eloquent witness to that desperate battle.

►Continue on the shady trail alongside El Camino Del Mar toward Point Lobos Avenue. A pair of short staircases drop you into the large Merrie Way parking lot. Circle the lot to the west, where another staircase drops steeply down toward the ruins of the Sutro Baths.

►Make sure your tour of the pools includes a visit to the overlook on the bluff to the north (right, as you face the Pacific). The vista is so vast that the ocean appears to spill off the curve of the earth, contained only by the Marin Headlands to the north and the Cliff House and Seal Rocks to the south.

►A traversing path leads up out of the baths to the south, depositing you on Point Lobos Avenue beside Louis' Restaurant, a fixture on Point Lobos for more than seventy-five years. Use the crosswalk to get across Point Lobos into the parking lot for Sutro Heights Park. The sidewalk that splits the lot leads onto a forested path that climbs onto the promenade encircling the park.

►At the small white gazebo, turn right and head toward the Pacific. The broad, gravel promenade is lined with palm trees, Monterey pines, eucalyptus, and fir. The park, with its gardens, crumbling statues, and ruins, radiates history. Adolph Sutro, mining engineer, oceanfront developer, and onetime mayor of San Francisco, built this hilltop retreat at the end of the nineteenth century.

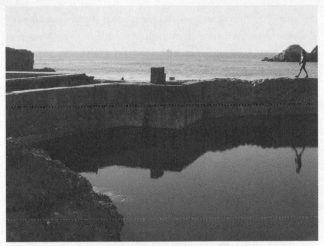
Water pools in the ruins of Sutro Baths, still and calm in contrast to the surf crashing on the other side of the walls.

▶The promenade continues around the perimeter of the park, along an overlook with a grand view of the Pacific Ocean. But the best view is arguably to the south, where you look down upon Ocean Beach, the sun-splashed apartments that stand on the former site of Playland at the Beach, and, even farther to the south, Fort Funston and the suburb of Pacifica.

▶Continue along the perimeter path to where the foundations for Sutro's mansion and garden overlook rise to the left. Take the rough steps that look as if they were carved out of the bedrock; these lead to the parapet, with its breathtaking views.

▶Descend from the parapet via any route you chose and continue to ramble along the promenade. As you complete the circuit, a broad path leads northeast toward Point Lobos Avenue. Bear right and follow the trail out between the two statues of lions that guard the entrance to the park.

▶Cross Point Lobos Avenue at the light and end your walk in the Merrie Way parking lot (5 miles).

OTHER DISTINCTIVE NEIGHBORHOODS

Walk 12: Pacific Heights and Japantown

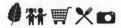

General location: North-central San Francisco

Special attractions: Shopping districts; cafes and restaurants; urban landscapes and varied architecture; a city park; a Japanese cultural center

Difficulty: Moderate. The route is hilly but almost entirely follows sidewalks.

Distance: 3.6 miles

Estimated time: 2 hours

Services: Restaurants, restrooms

Restrictions: Not wheelchair accessible. A few hills are so steep that steps have been added to make climbing easier; there are a few dirt pathways in Lafayette Park. Dogs must be leashed (except in Lafayette Park's dog-run area) and their droppings picked up.

For more information: The San Francisco Travel Association, 900 Market St., Hallidie Plaza, San Francisco, CA 94102-2804; (415) 391-2000; sanfrancisco.travel

Getting started: Begin at the corner of Union and Buchanan Streets. GPS: N37 47.857' / W122 25.930'

(1) From the intersection of Market, Ninth, Hayes, and Larkin Streets near the Civic Center, veer left onto Hayes and go 3 blocks. Turn right onto Franklin Street and go about 1.5 miles to Union Street. Turn left onto Union and go 4 blocks to Buchanan.

(2) From the Golden Gate Bridge, continue south on US 101 / Presidio Parkway, staying right onto Lombard Street. Drive 7 blocks on Lombard Street, turn right onto Buchanan Street, and go 3 blocks to Union Street. On-street parking is extremely scarce in this neighborhood. The two garages closest to the start of this walk are California Parking between Laguna and Buchanan Streets, and Union Street Plaza at 2001 Union between Buchanan and Webster Streets.

Public transportation: San Francisco Municipal Railway (Muni) buses run along Union Street. Contact Muni for information about schedules, fares, and accessibility (sfmta .com, tripplanner.transit.511.org).

Overview: This pleasant walk leads through the eastern half of one of San Francisco's most affluent, mansion-studded neighborhoods, as well as through appealing shopping areas and into the center of Japantown.

The walk begins in Cow Hollow and climbs almost immediately into Pacific Heights, two neighborhoods that radiate urbanity. The residences are perfectly manicured, the restaurants are upscale, and the boutiques are first-class (even the consignment shops). On the steep and serene streets of Pacific Heights, you will encounter astonishing feats of architecture, from private Victorian mansions to elegant neoclassical apartment houses. Affluence breeds good shopping, and the two lively retail streets on this walk—Union and Fillmore—cater to discriminating tastes. You will also find plenty of great places to eat, from espresso and pastry to *banh mi*.

The walk takes on another flavor when it enters Japantown. Many of San Francisco's Japanese citizens settled here, in the city's Western Addition, after the 1906 earthquake and fire. Today, the East and West Japan Center Malls (formerly the Japanese Cultural and Trade Center), with their many shops and restaurants, serve as a focal point for the city's thriving Japanese community.

San Francisco firefighters managed to stop the great fire of 1906 at Van Ness Avenue, thus preserving many of the beautiful Victorian homes—large and small—of the Western Addition and Pacific Heights. Some of the city's finest restored Victorians are found on the steep streets that run between the two districts.

You'll pass through little Lafayette Park at the highest point in Pacific Heights, a pocket of palm trees and rolling lawn amid concrete and asphalt. Soak up a little nature, then descend back to Union Street and into the urban fray.

The Walk

▶Start at the corner of Union and Buchanan Streets, facing west. Walk along Union for 1 block to Webster Street. This stretch of Union Street (between Gough and Steiner Streets) is one of San Francisco's chic shopping districts, crowded with antiques stores, interior design salons, clothing boutiques, and art emporiums, plus an enticing array of restaurants, bakeries, and coffeehouses.

▸ Turn right onto Webster and go 1 block to the corner of Webster and Filbert, where you can check out a San Francisco landmark at 2963 Webster. Built for the Vedanta Society in 1905 by architect Joseph Leonard, this East-meets-West extravaganza, with its distinctive Asian appurtenances mixed with Victorian gingerbread, adds flash to an otherwise sedate architectural setting.

▸ Walk back up Webster to Union. Cross Union and climb 3 blocks up Webster to Broadway. Between Vallejo and Broadway, steps cut into the sidewalk help mitigate Webster's steepness. The climb takes you into the tony residential district known as Pacific Heights, with spectacular mansions and elegant apartment houses in a variety of architectural styles lining the relatively quiet boulevards.

▸ Turn right onto Broadway and walk 1 block to Fillmore Street, passing the Schools of the Sacred Heart, housed in three handsome historic mansions at 2200, 2222, and 2252 Broadway. The western section of Pacific Heights, reached by continuing west on Broadway, encompasses extraordinarily expensive homes and mansions, many on the scale of the ones you've already passed. Make a note to return another day to explore the area bounded by Broadway, Jackson, Fillmore, and Lyon Streets. From the corner of Fillmore and Lyon, you can descend the rather grand Lyon Street steps to return to Union Street. Be sure to take in the sweeping views of the bay from the top of the hill.

▸ Turn left onto Fillmore and walk downhill through this delightful shopping district for 8 blocks. All manner of specialty stores, from vintage-clothing boutiques to French

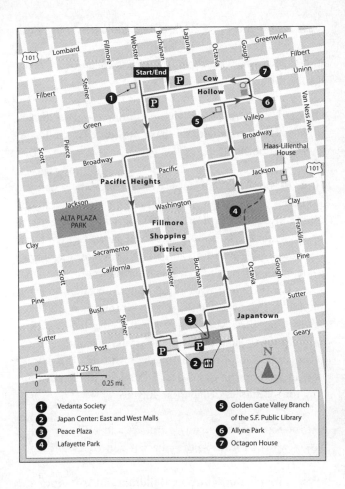

Start/End

Lombard

101

Filbert

Green

Broadway

Pacific Heights

Jackson

ALTA PLAZA
PARK

Sacramento

California

Pine

Bush

Sutter

Post

Fillmore
Steiner
Pierce
Scott

Webster
Buchanan
Laguna
Octavia
Gough
Greenwich

Filbert
Union
Cow
Hollow
Vallejo
Broadway
Haas-Lilienthal
House
Jackson
101
Clay
Franklin
Pine
Gough
Octavia
Sutter
Geary
Van Ness Ave.

Pacific

Washington

Fillmore
Shopping
District

Webster
Buchanan

Clay

Scott

Steiner

Japantown

Peace Plaza

Lafayette Park

P

P

P

P

6

7

5

4

3

2

1

N

0   0.25 km.
0   0.25 mi.

1	Vedanta Society	5	Golden Gate Valley Branch
2	Japan Center: East and West Malls		of the S.F. Public Library
3	Peace Plaza	6	Allyne Park
4	Lafayette Park	7	Octagon House

patisseries, bodegas to purveyors of high-end furniture, open onto the tree-lined sidewalk.

▶Just before you cross Bush Street, look left along Bush to the row of Victorians at numbers 2115, 2117, 2119, and 2121 Bush, with their false fronts elegantly outlined against the sky.

▶Proceed 2 more blocks along Fillmore to Post Street, cross Post, and turn left. You have now entered the Japantown neighborhood.

▶Just beyond the entrance to the Sundance Cinema multiplex of theaters, you will find the entrance to the Kinokuniya Building (1825 Post), part of East and West Japan Center Malls, also known as the Japan Center. Enter the Kinokuniya Building and ascend its central stairway. Some of the center's restaurants offer the traditional Japanese style of dining, with guests seated on tatami mats at low tables. Many offer sushi or a simple menu of large bowls of noodles. Most of the Japan Center's shops focus on traditional Japanese arts and crafts: Japanese prints, paper lamps, kimonos, and antique furniture. The grocery store located on the ground level bustles with locals shopping for the staples of Japanese cuisine.

▶At the top of the stairway, turn left and walk through a passageway that leads to the adjacent Kintetsu Building.

▶Pass through the Kintetsu Building and exit onto the open-air Peace Plaza, with the Peace Pagoda towering above. The multitiered pagoda was presented in friendship

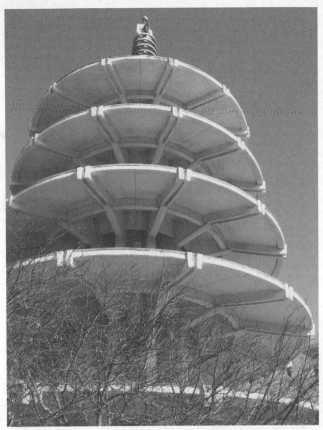

The Peace Pagoda marks the center of San Francisco's Japantown.

to the people of the United States by the people of Japan in 1968.

▶Exit the Peace Plaza onto Post Street. Cross Post and walk 1 block (a block of Buchanan Street) down a walking mall bordered by shops and restaurants housed in buildings with Japanese-inspired architecture. If you managed not to sit down for a meal in the Japan Center, the outdoor mall offers you plenty of second chances.

▸At the corner of Sutter and Buchanan Streets, cross Sutter, turn right, and walk 1 block up Sutter to Laguna Street. Take a left onto Laguna and head uphill through a famous and photogenic group of Victorian homes. Continue up Laguna 3 blocks to California Street.

▸Take a right onto California. Check out the spectacular row of Victorians—handsomely painted and each different from the next—across the street.

▸At the corner of California and Octavia Streets, turn left, crossing California and continuing up Octavia for 1 block. Check out the enormous house on the corner of California and Octavia, with its tower and cupola. Handsome mansions like this one—and many of the stylish apartment buildings in the neighborhood—underscore the wealth and restraint of the Pacific Heights district.

▸Octavia Street runs into Lafayette Park at Sacramento Street. Cross Sacramento and pass between the set of palm trees flanking the entrance to the park. Continue straight ahead, up to the crest of the park, which is crowned in cypress, eucalyptus, and palm trees. Lafayette Park is popular with dog lovers; it has an official dog-run area where Rover can roam off-leash.

▶At the crown of the hill, take the path to the right. With the city out of sight, you might be able to convince yourself you are in the countryside instead of in a 4-block park surrounded by a dense urban neighborhood. Barking dogs and the laughter of children wafting up from the playground add to the ambience.

▶Head toward the northeastern corner of the park, to the intersection of Washington and Gough Streets. As the city makes its presence known again, you'll see a row of striking Queen Anne homes on Gough Street, off to the right.

▶Descend the steps leading out of the park, turn left, and walk 1 block along Washington. Enormous private residences—some with parklike grounds, an extreme luxury in this crowded city—line the block. Note also the grand rose-colored apartment building at 2006 Washington, with its spectacular entranceway and formal garden. The immense French-style mansion at 2080 Washington was built by George Applegarth, the architect who also designed the Palace of the Legion of Honor in Lincoln Park.

▶Turn right onto Octavia and descend 1 block through a pleasant oasis of greenery alongside the quiet, brick-paved street.

▶At the corner of Octavia and Jackson, take in the view of the bay, including Fort Mason, Alcatraz, and Angel Island. Then turn left onto Jackson.

THE HAAS-LILIENTHAL HOUSE

There are Victorians in San Francisco . . . and then there are Victorians. Pacific Heights has its share, including the extraordinary Haas-Lilienthal House. Situated at 2007 Franklin St. (about 2 blocks northeast of Lafayette Park and an easy addition to the Pacific Heights walk), this historic Queen Anne functions as a museum run by SF Heritage (sfheritage .org), the only Victorian in the city that is open to the public for docent-led tours.

The Haas-Lilienthal House was built in 1886. Like its neighbors throughout Pacific Heights, it escaped the 1906 fire because the city's fire brigades were able to stop the conflagration at Van Ness Avenue. The house's beautifully preserved interior—many of

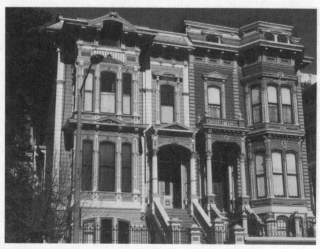

Classic San Francisco Victorians line the streets of Pacific Heights.

the furnishings are original—reflects the taste of William Haas and his descendants, including daughter Alice Lilienthal, whose heirs donated the home to the Foundation for San Francisco's Architectural Heritage after her death in 1972. Though this house cost nearly $20,000 to build, a hefty price in its day, other San Francisco mansions of the same period topped the $1 million mark, a testimony to the extraordinary wealth this city generated during the nineteenth century.

▶At the corner of Jackson and Laguna, cross Jackson and descend the hill on Laguna for 1 block to Pacific.

▶Cross Pacific and turn right, noting the Victorians at 2023, 2021, and 2019 Pacific and the wonderful Queen Anne—with its gorgeous curved windows—at 2000 Pacific, on the corner of Octavia and Pacific. This Queen Anne sports a formal garden in its front yard, complete with roses and perfectly trimmed hedges.

▶Turn left onto Octavia, descending the hill for 3 blocks and passing more fine Victorians.

▶At the corner of Octavia and Green Streets, turn left and walk one-quarter block on Green to look at the Golden Gate Valley branch of the San Francisco Public Library, the unusual neoclassical building at 1801 Green.

▶Return to the corner of Octavia and Green and continue on Green 1 block to Gough Street.

▸Turn left onto Gough and descend 1 block to Union Street. Pass Allyne Park, a compact pocket of greenery with lawn and shade trees, and then the Octagon House at 2645 Gough. The Octagon House, built in 1861, followed on the ideas of Orson Fowler, who proposed that octagonal houses were conducive to better, more healthful living. Run as a museum, listed on the National Register of Historic Places, and open to the public on a limited basis, the Octagon is run by the National Society of Colonial Dames (nscda.org/museums2/ca-octagonhouse .html). Another octagonal house, used as a private residence, can be found on Russian Hill.

▸Turn left onto Union and walk 3 blocks to the corner of Union and Buchanan and the end of this walk.

Walk 13: The Castro District and Noe Valley

🏢🛒✕

General location: In central San Francisco, below Twin Peaks, about 2 miles southwest of Union Square

Special attractions: Urban landscapes and vistas; neighborhood shopping districts, cafes, and restaurants; varied architecture; hill climbing

Difficulty: Strenuous, with steep hills and stairways, but entirely on sidewalks

Distance: 4.1 miles

Estimated time: 2.5 hours

Services: Restaurants, restrooms

Restrictions: Not wheelchair accessible. Dogs must be leashed and their droppings picked up.

For more information: The San Francisco Travel Association, 900 Market St., Hallidie Plaza, San Francisco, CA 94102-2804; (415) 391-2000; sanfrancisco.travel

Getting started: This walk begins at Harvey Milk Plaza, located at the southwest corner of the intersection of Market, Castro, and 17th Streets, 2 miles southwest of downtown San Francisco. GPS: N37 45.746' / W122 26.123'

(1) From the intersection of Ninth, Market, Hayes, and Larkin Streets, turn left onto Market and go 1.5 miles to the intersection of Market with Castro and 17th Streets.

(2) From the Golden Gate Bridge, continue south on US 101 / Presidio Parkway, staying right onto Lombard Street. Drive 1 block on Lombard Street and turn right onto Divisadero Street. Drive 2 miles to where Divisadero

turns into Castro Street, and then go another 0.5 mile on Castro to the intersection of Castro, Market, and 17th Streets.

On-street parking in this neighborhood is scarce and metered/time-restricted. Limited parking is available at Market and Noe Center Public Parking on Noe Street. Your best bet: Leave the car behind and take a taxi or public transportation to the start of the walk.

Public transportation: San Francisco Municipal Railway (Muni) streetcar line F, as well as buses and Muni Metro lines, all stop at Market and Castro Streets. Contact Muni for information about schedules, fares, and accessibility (sfmta.com, tripplanner.transit.511.org).

Overview: This invigorating walk takes you into three distinctive San Francisco neighborhoods. From the humble and historic Harvey Milk Plaza on the corner of Castro and Market Streets, climb into the Upper Castro and lower Twin Peaks residential areas. The garden-lined and very steep Vulcan Street stairs help you gain altitude in a neighborhood noted for its eclectic mix of architectural styles and maze of curvy streets—quite unlike the grid that overlays the rest of San Francisco. The neighborhood is rarely visited by tourists, so you may find yourself marvelously alone.

Drop into Noe Valley, one of San Francisco's most fashionable neighborhoods. Tucked between hills that separate the district from downtown and the Castro, Noe Valley has a village flair, with trendy restaurants and coffee shops sporting lines that wind out the doors and fashionable boutiques displaying their wares and services along 24th Street.

From Noe Valley, climb over the hill and into the lower Castro District, which, unlike the Upper Castro, is rarely quiet. The Castro, with its overwhelmingly gay population, is integral to San Francisco's identity. San Franciscans celebrate, take pride in, and wholeheartedly accept the city's diversity, which encompasses every color of the rainbow.

End the walk as you began it, in Harvey Milk Plaza next to the historic Castro Theatre. Harvey Milk—San Francisco's first openly gay city supervisor—was tragically assassinated, along with the city's mayor, George Moscone, on November 27, 1978.

The Walk

▸Start at Harvey Milk Plaza, the small brick-paved plaza located at the three-way intersection of Market, Castro, and 17th Streets. The main entrance to the Castro/Market Muni Metro station is here; escalators lead from the plaza down to the underground station.

▸Cross Market Street at the light. Turn left onto the sidewalk that parallels 17th Street, which is not well marked at this point. As you continue up the sidewalk, you'll pass a street sign confirming that you are, indeed, on 17th. Pass a few Victorians, some painted in the purples and greens of peacocks, others in more muted tones.

▸Walk uphill on 17th for 4 blocks to Ord Street. The last 2 blocks are fairly steep.

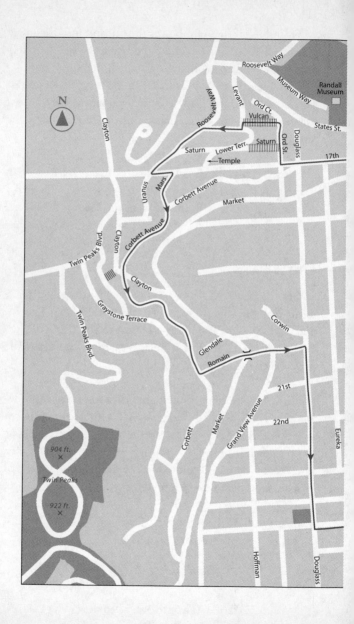

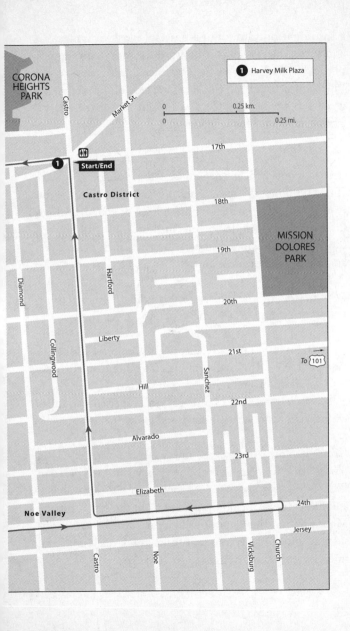

CORONA
HEIGHTS
PARK

Market St.

Castro

1 Harvey Milk Plaza

0   0.25 km.
0   0.25 mi.

17th

1 Start/End

Castro District

18th

MISSION
DOLORES
PARK

19th

Hartford

Diamond

20th

Collingwood

Liberty

21st

To 101

Sanchez

Hill

22nd

Alvarado

23rd

Elizabeth

24th

Noe Valley

Jersey

Castro

Noe

Vicksburg

Church

▸Turn right on Ord, onto a peaceful block of bungalows and Victorians. Follow Ord toward the rocky outcropping of Corona Heights, past the Saturn Street stairs, to the Vulcan Street stairs on the left-hand side of the street. The grasslands of the tiny Corona Heights city park boast a great wildflower bloom in season.

▸Turn left onto the Vulcan Street stairs and climb the steps—about 215 in all—to the top. When you have climbed about 55 steps, a second stairway branches off to the left. Stay on the right-hand set of stairs. Gardens flourish in this secluded ravine, lush with colorful flowers, fragrant herbs, bamboo hedges, berry bushes, palm trees, and a variety of exotic plants.

▸At the top of the Vulcan Street stairs, turn left onto Levant Street and go a partial block to Lower Terrace.

▸Turn right onto Lower Terrace and walk uphill 1 block to Roosevelt Way. The houses along this quiet stretch show-case a variety of architectural styles, from Mission bungalows to Victorians to standard San Francisco–style flats with the requisite bay windows and garage below.

▸Turn left onto Roosevelt and walk 2 mercifully level blocks back to 17th Street. The grassy summits of Twin Peaks—904 feet and 922 feet above sea level—rise ahead, and Sutro Tower juts like a trident from the top of nearby Mount Sutro. This enormous antenna, which many consider an appalling eyesore, transmits radio, television, and microwave signals throughout the Bay Area.

▶Cross 17th Street at the stop sign. There is a small grocery on this corner, your last chance to buy refreshments until you reach Noe Valley, about 1 mile farther on.

▶Turn left onto 17th and walk downhill 1 short block to Mars Street.

▶Turn right onto Mars—how lucky you would be to say you live on Mars, which turns out to be quite civilized. Walk 1 block to Corbett Avenue, where Mars dead-ends.

▶Cross Corbett, turn right, and walk uphill along Corbett. On your left, near the street sign marking the intersection of Mono and Corbett Avenue, pass Corbett Slope Community Park, which dives down the hillside. The bulk of the park is behind a fence, with no obvious place to sit and rest, but a half-block farther on, you'll find a bench at tiny Al's Park.

▶Where Corbett meets Clayton Street (1.2 miles), turn left and walk along Clayton a short distance to the crosswalk. Cross the street and continue straight ahead on the continuation of Corbett. The narrow roadway winds upward through the lower part of Twin Peaks, its 1960s multiunit structures built to take advantage of spectacular views of the city and the bay. Peek through the fences to catch glimpses of the Noe Valley, downtown San Francisco, and the Mission District.

▶When you reach Romain Street (1.5 miles), turn left onto Romain and walk downhill 1 block, passing a series of colorful Spanish-style stucco bungalows. Built in the

1930s, the tiny front gardens of these homes are planted with native wildflowers and succulents.

▸At the bottom of the block, cross Market Street via the pedestrian bridge. From the bridge take in the sweeping views of downtown San Francisco and the East Bay. A spiral ramp leads down off the bridge and onto the next block of Romain.

▸Continue walking downhill on Romain for 2 blocks. Where Romain collides with Douglass Street, descend a flight of stairs onto Douglass and turn right.

▸Follow Douglass Street for 6 blocks to 24th Street. Glance up and down 23rd Street to see clusters of classic San Francisco Victorians. Dogs and children gather in the park at Noe Valley Courts, which occupies the block between Elizabeth and 24th Streets.

▸Turn left onto 24th Street and walk 5 blocks to Church Street, enjoying the color, smell, and buoyancy of Noe Valley's busy neighborhood shopping area. The blocks are lined with cafes and restaurants, bookstores and bakeries, gourmet food shops, wine merchants, and other small businesses. Although a couple of chain coffeehouses make appearances on the street, most of Noe Valley's businesses are one-of-a-kind and are housed in old Victorians. If you need a pick-me-up after your hill-climbing, this is just the place.

▸At Church Street cross to the opposite side of 24th Street and walk back 3 blocks to Castro Street (3.2 miles).

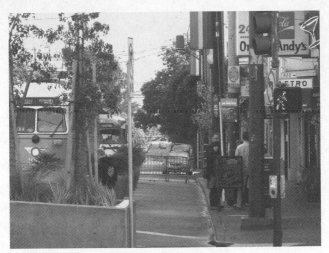
Vintage streetcars serve the Castro District.

▸Turn right onto Castro and walk 3 steep blocks to Alvarado Street at the crest of the hill. Some beautifully painted and lovingly maintained Victorians line this stretch of Castro. It's worth looking (or walking) up and down the cross streets for even more Victorian gazing.

▸Descend 6 blocks on Castro to 19th Street. This is the heart of the Castro, one of the best-known gay neighborhoods in the United States. The Castro's bustling commercial district starts at 18th Street and continues up toward Harvey Milk Plaza. Businesses include vintage-clothing stores, antiques emporiums, and home-furnishing stores, as well as cafes, bars, and restaurants. The striking neon sign for the Castro Theatre, a neighborhood landmark dating back to 1922 and one of the last grand movie theaters still operating in San Francisco, rises above it all. The theater is known for showing excellent modern, foreign, cult, and classic movies, and—keeping alive a venerable cinematic tradition—features music from its Wurlitzer pipe organ.

▶Continue past the Castro Theatre to the corner of 17th, Castro, and Market Streets. Cross Castro to return to Harvey Milk Plaza and the end of this walk.

Walk 14: Mission Murals

♿ 🏢 👪 🛒 ✗ 📷

General location: In central San Francisco off Mission Street, about 2.5 miles south of Union Square

Special attractions: Colorful murals; distinctive neighborhood; restaurants

Difficulty: Easy, flat, and entirely on sidewalks

Distance: 2.0 miles

Estimated time: 1 hour

Services: Restaurants

Restrictions: Wheelchair accessible. Dogs must be leashed and their droppings picked up. The murals in this neighborhood are copyrighted works of art. Feel free to photograph them for your personal use, but note that photos of the murals cannot be reproduced except with written permission from the muralist(s). If you wish to obtain permission, call Precita Eyes Mural Arts Center.

For more information: The San Francisco Travel Association, 900 Market St., Hallidie Plaza, San Francisco, CA 94102-2804; (415) 391-2000; sanfrancisco.travel. Precita Eyes Mural Arts Center, 2981 24th St., San Francisco, CA 94110; (415) 285-2287; precitaeyes.org.

Getting started: This walk begins at the corner of Mission and 24th Streets. GPS: N37 45.130' / W122 25.095'

(1) From the intersection of Ninth and Howard Streets (2 blocks south of the intersection of Market, Ninth, Larkin, and Hayes Streets), drive southwest on Howard for 4 blocks until Howard merges into South Van Ness Avenue. Continue southward on South Van Ness for 1.25 miles to

24th Street. Turn right onto 24th Street, and go 2 blocks to Mission Street.

(2) From the Golden Gate Bridge, continue south on US 101/Presidio Parkway, staying right onto Lombard Street. Drive about 1 mile on Lombard Street to Van Ness Avenue. Turn right onto Van Ness and drive 1.75 miles to Market Street. Cross Market and continue on South Van Ness for 1.5 miles. Turn right onto 24th Street and go 2 blocks to Mission Street.

There are no parking garages close by, but on-street parking is available on 24th and its side streets, and a tiny outdoor parking lot (metered) is located on 24th at Lilac Street.

Public transportation: Several San Francisco Municipal Railway (Muni) bus routes, as well as trains of the Bay Area Rapid Transit (BART) system, stop at 24th and Mission Streets. Contact Muni (sfmta.com, tripplanner .transit.511.org) or BART (bart.gov) for schedules, fares, and accessibility.

Overview: The neighborhood surrounding 24th Street in the Mission District has a distinctly Latin feel. This is a working-class community: The sidewalks are crowded with shoppers, families walking hand in hand, and clusters of old-timers sharing stories on street corner benches. The tree-lined stretch of 24th between Mission and York Streets overflows with vegetable and grocery stores, *panaderias* (bakeries), restaurants, *carnicerias* (meat markets), art galleries, and numerous gift shops.

And 24th Street has something that no other neighborhood in the city offers: an amazing array of beautiful, well-crafted, and thought-provoking murals depicting themes of importance to the artists and local residents. There are more than eighty murals in the Mission District, and this walk samples a representative group of them. Branch off on other streets—down Mission, into the surrounding neighborhood—and you'll see others: bright frescos over doorways, vibrant garage doors, panels flanking shops. What's remarkable is that, while vacant walls may be tagged with graffiti, especially if you wander into more run-down areas of the Mission, the murals remain largely untouched, a hopeful display of respect for the pride of a community.

The Walk

▶Start at the corner of 24th and Mission Streets, in front of the McDonald's restaurant on the southeast corner. This is probably the only McDonald's in the world decorated with a vibrant mural created by neighborhood kids. Stroll east into the 24th Street business district. An abundance of color enlivens the boulevard aside from the murals . . . but the murals are everywhere, usually several to a block on both sides of the street. No worries about missing anything; the sidewalks are typically crowded enough that you'll be moving slowly.

▶Walk 5.5 blocks to Balmy Alley, a block-long lane that's more of a pedestrian walkway. Turn right into the alley, which is decorated with back-to-back murals on both sides, the highest concentration in the Mission. Above the murals the buildings are workaday, with laundry fluttering off balconies and music emanating from open kitchen windows. At the end of the alley, turn around and walk back to 24th Street.

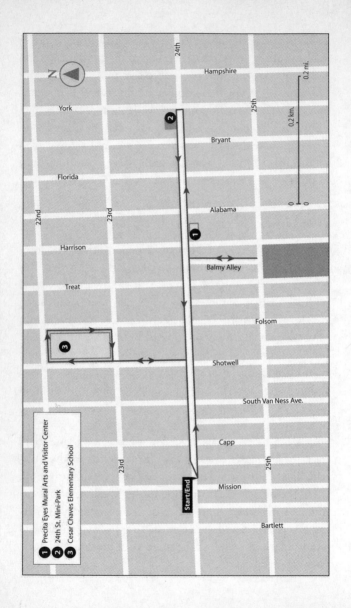

►Turn right onto 24th Street and walk for one-half block to Harrison Street. On this corner, at La Gallinita Belmar Meat Market, is a mural of two mythic Mexican figures: Popocatépetl, a warrior, and Ixtaccihuatl, the daughter of the emperor. Their love was ill-fated, and as Ixtaccihuatl lay dying, Popocatépetl swept her away. Transformed into a mountain and a volcano, the lovers lie side by side outside Mexico City, together forever. These legendary figures appear in many Mission murals.

►Continue on 24th Street one-half block to the Precita Eyes Mural Arts and Visitor Center (precitaeyes.org) at 2981 24th St. The center conducts mural tours and workshops, and the friendly staff can also provide Mission District cultural and business information. Feel free to stop in to look at the mural-covered walls, check out the colorful mural postcards, or pick up a map that identifies the eighty-four murals in the Mission District.

►Continue on 24th another half block to Alabama Street. Look up high on the wall of the Mexican bakery on this corner, which is adorned with trompe l'oeil roof tiles, as well as the heroic figures painted on its exterior walls.

►Continue on 24th for one-half block to the mural on the building that houses the Modern Times Bookstore Collective, *A Bountiful Harvest*. China Books and Periodicals commissioned this mural in the style of Chinese social realism, except that the classic harvest scene depicts people of many races.

THE MURALS OF BALMY ALLEY

The murals on the back fences and garage doors of this quiet alley have been created over five decades. Whether dimmed by rain, sun, and fog or vibrant and new, these works of art are provocative and inspirational, sometimes lighthearted, and reflective of Latino cultural pride and San Francisco's diverse cultural heritage. What you'll see here from year to year is an evolution, from panels honoring cultural icons like the great Mexican muralist Diego Rivera (one of the founders of the Mexican mural movement) and his wife, painter Frida Kahlo, to a celebration of low-rider culture, to a portrait of Michael Jackson, to a missing page from Maurice Sendak's *Where the Wild Things Are*. . . . Other murals on Balmy Alley deal with painful subjects, such as mothers holding photos of family members "disappeared" by death squads, statements about Central American politics and history, memorials to those who have died of AIDS or worked with those victims, and things falling apart. Contact the Precita Eyes Mural Arts Center (precita eyes.org) to take a tour of Balmy Alley and learn more about the Mission murals.

▶Continue on 24th another half block to Florida Street. The powerful mural *500 Años de Resistencia* ("500 Years of Resistance"), painted by Isaías Mata, spreads across two faces of St. Peter's Church. Completed in 1993, this mural depicts the survival of native cultures despite the invasion of the American continents by Europeans.

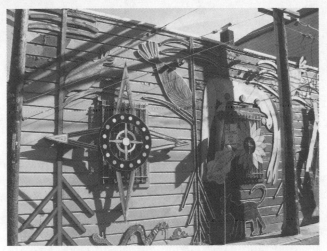

The murals of Balmy Alley encapsulate the artistic energies that spill out onto the Mission District's 24th Street. This is *Five Sacred Colors of Corn* (copyright 1991 Susan Kelk Cervantes).

▶Continue on 24th 1 block to Bryant. Galeria de la Raza is on this corner. Founded in 1970, Galeria de la Raza is one of the oldest Latino arts organizations in the United States. It offers art exhibitions, multimedia presentations, and educational activities related to Chicano/Latino art.

▶Continue on 24th for 1 block to York Street. The St. Francis Fountain and Candy Store has been on this corner since 1918. This old-time family-run soda fountain is known for its handmade ice cream and candy.

▶Cross 24th to the opposite side, and look across York at the powerful mural on the side of SF Taqueria. *La Llorona's Sacred Waters* was created in 2004 by Juana Alicia, replacing her 1983 mural *Las Lechugueras*, which paid tribute to Mexican-American women farmworkers. Alicia's work was inspired by women's environmental struggles, and evokes the myth of a Mexican mother who drowned her children and was condemned to weep for them.

▶ Walk back one-half block on 24th toward Mission Street. The 24th Street Mini-Park is midblock, between York and Bryant Streets This park's murals, created between 1974 and 1990, were designed to teach children in the community about their Latin American heritage. A tiled serpentine play structure, inspired by the Mexican god Quetzalcoatl, winds through the park, and benches allow visitors to rest and contemplate the amazing art that surrounds them.

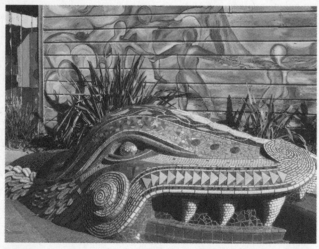

Children can play on a mosaic serpent in the 24th Street Mini-Park.

▶Continue 1.5 blocks to Florida Street and La Palma Market, one of the last places in the Mission selling handmade tortillas. The mural on the Florida Street side of the market is an eye-catching advertisement for those tortillas.

▶Continue 5 blocks on 24th to Shotwell Street. Turn right onto Shotwell.

▶Go 2 blocks on Shotwell to 22nd Street, passing the front entrance of the Cesar Chavez Elementary School. This school is covered with some of the most beautiful murals in the Mission, and this loop allows you to see all four sides.

▶Turn right onto 22nd, go 1 block to Folsom, turn right, and walk 1 block on Folsom. Walking back toward 24th on Folsom takes you past the school playground, which is dominated by the larger-than-life mural called *Si Se Puede* ("Yes We Can"). Painted in vibrant reds, blues, yellows, and greens, this mural weaves in and out among the classroom windows, and is anchored by a two-story portrait of Cesar Chavez—California's great farmworker/organizer—over the school doors.

▶Turn right onto 23rd Street and walk 1 block to Shotwell Street.

▶Turn left onto Shotwell and go 1 block to 24th.

▶Turn right onto 24th and walk 3 blocks to the corner of Mission and 24th and the end of this walk.

PARKLANDS

Walk 15: Golden Gate Park

🍃 👫 ✕ 📷

General location: In central San Francisco, about 3 miles west of Union Square

Special attractions: An expansive park with abundant walking paths; art and science museums; botanical gardens; boating

Difficulty: Easy

Distance: 3.0 miles

Estimated time: 1.5 hours

Services: Parking, restrooms, snack bar, bicycle and Segway rentals, boat rentals

Restrictions: Not wheelchair accessible. Dogs must be leashed and their droppings picked up. John F. Kennedy Drive is closed to auto traffic for half days on Sat and all day Sun (no parking permitted alongside the road either) from Stanyan Street to Park Presidio.

For more information: The San Francisco Travel Association, 900 Market St., Hallidie Plaza, San Francisco, CA 94102-2804; (415) 391-2000; sanfrancisco.travel. Golden Gate Park, golden-gate-park.com.

Getting started: This walk begins in front of the Conservatory of Flowers, near the eastern edge of Golden Gate Park. GPS: N37 46.333' / W122 27.616'

(1) From I-80 westbound and/or US 101 northbound, follow US 101 north to the Fell/Laguna exit. Drive about

1.5 miles west on Fell Street. Fell turns into John F. Kennedy Drive, one of Golden Gate Park's main roadways, at Stanyon Street. Continue 0.25 mile on John F. Kennedy Drive to the Conservatory of Flowers.

(2) From the San Francisco Peninsula, take I-280 northbound to the Golden Gate Bridge / 19th Avenue exit, just beyond Daly City (stay in the left-hand lanes of the freeway). Continue on CA 1 northbound for almost 5 miles, following Junipero Serra Boulevard, 19th Avenue, and Park Presidio through Golden Gate Park. On the northern boundary of the park, turn right onto Fulton Street, go 3.5 blocks, and turn right onto 10th Avenue. At the next stop sign, turn left onto John F. Kennedy Drive and go 0.5 mile to the Conservatory of Flowers.

(3) From the Golden Gate Bridge, stay right on the Park Presidio / 19th Avenue off-ramp and drive about 2 miles south on Park Presidio Boulevard. One block before Golden Gate Park's northern boundary, turn right onto Cabrillo Street, and then make an immediate left turn onto 14th Avenue. Drive 1 block and turn left onto Fulton Street. Cross Park Presidio and continue on Fulton for 3.5 blocks. Turn right onto 10th Avenue. At the next stop sign, turn left onto John F. Kennedy Drive and go 0.5 mile to the Conservatory of Flowers.

Parking is available along John F. Kennedy Drive; try to get as close as possible to the Conservatory of Flowers, an unmistakable and grand white glass-and-wood structure.

Public transportation: A number of San Francisco Municipal Railway (Muni) buses stop within 1 to 5 blocks of McLaren Lodge, administrative headquarters for San Francisco's recreation and parks department, which oversees Golden Gate Park. Contact Muni (sfmta.com, tripplanner

.transit.511.org) for schedules, fares, and accessibility. A park shuttle runs on Sat, Sun, and major holidays; a fee is charged.

Overview: Golden Gate Park—like Fisherman's Wharf, Chinatown, and the Golden Gate Bridge—is integral to San Francisco's identity. The bridge is the gateway, the wharf and Chinatown embody crucial aspects of the city's cultural identity, and the park is San Francisco's "plaza," it's common ground, a place to celebrate and to find peace, to learn, to wander.

In the 1,017 acres of Golden Gate Park—it is 3 miles long and a handful of blocks wide, a linear swipe of green space linking city streets to Ocean Beach—you can pursue nearly every outdoor activity, from in-line skating and lawn bowling to fly casting and horseback riding. You can wander through redwood groves, rhododendron dells, botanical gardens, and a Japanese tea garden. You can row a boat or dance to reggae or run for miles on paths that loop through meadow and woodland. You can gaze at masterpieces of European and Asian art, learn about the world's oceans, and picnic in grassy meadows.

Golden Gate Park had inauspicious beginnings, at least for an open space now known for its magnificent gardens and towering trees. First chosen as the site for a great public park in the 1860s, the acreage was little more than sand dunes whipped by ocean winds. Civil engineer William Hammond Hall was the park's designer and first superintendent. In addition to surveying the park, he began the long process of turning a sandy wasteland into a luxuriant parkland, stabilizing the dunes by planting lupine, barley, and beach grasses imported from France. In those early years, more than 200,000 trees were planted. Slowly, laboriously, Golden Gate Park was transformed.

The park's second hero, Scottish garden designer John McLaren, carried on in Hall's spirit over a career that spanned nearly sixty years, overseeing the creation of many of the park features that remain on the ground today.

This walk leads to some of the park's signature attractions, including the Conservatory of Flowers, the museums surrounding the Music Concourse, the San Francisco Botanical Gardens, and tranquil Stow Lake. These are what you might call the park's "main events," but there is much more to see and explore. With each visit you can rediscover a favorite place or encounter something new and different. The park extends an open invitation to return again, and again.

The Walk

▸Start in front of the Conservatory of Flowers. A Victorian marvel of wood and glass built in 1878, the conservatory is the oldest building in Golden Gate Park. The building was heavily damaged by a winter storm in 1995, but a $25 million restoration resulted in a grand reopening in 2003. The conservatory now houses both permanent and rotating horticultural exhibits, its glass walls protecting exotic orchids, bromeliads, ferns, aquatic plants, potted plants . . . too many to name. The conservatory is open Tues through Sun from 10 a.m. to 4:30 p.m.; a fee is charged. Call (415) 666-7001 for more information.

▸Once you have finished exploring the conservatory and the formal plantings that surround it, use the pedestrian

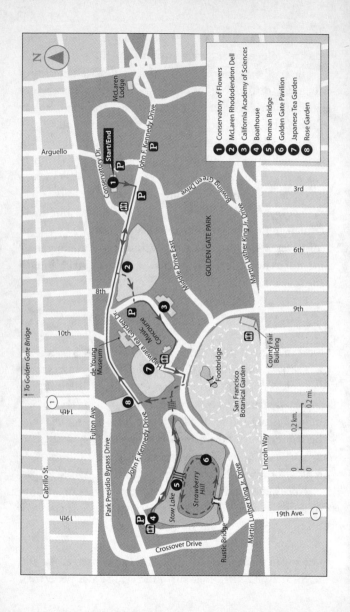

N

McLaren Lodge

Arguello

Start/End

Conservatory Dr.

John F. Kennedy Drive

P

P

1

Bowling Green Drive

3rd

6th

9th

GOLDEN GATE PARK

Martin Luther King Jr. Drive

2

Middle Drive East

8th

P

3

10th

de Young Museum

Music Concourse

Japanese Tea Garden Dr.

7

Footbridge

County Fair Building

San Francisco Botanical Garden

14th

To Golden Gate Bridge

1

Fulton Ave.

Park Presidio Bypass Drive

8

John F. Kennedy Drive

Lincoln Way

Cabrillo St.

16th

P

4

Stow Lake

5

6

Strawberry Hill

19th Ave.

1

Rustic Bridge

Crossover Drive

Martin Luther King Jr. Drive

0   0.2 km.

0   0.2 mi.

1. Conservatory of Flowers
2. McLaren Rhododendron Dell
3. California Academy of Sciences
4. Boathouse
5. Roman Bridge
6. Golden Gate Pavilion
7. Japanese Tea Garden
8. Rose Garden

tunnel that runs under John F. Kennedy Drive to get to the paved path on the far side of the roadway. Head right on the paved path alongside the busy drive.

▸A large wooden sign suspended over the path marks the entrance into the John McLaren Rhododendron Dell (0.4 mile). Turn left into the dell, onto the broad paved path and into a verdant grove. The dell is lush with agapanthus, rhododendron bushes, and expanses of raspberries.

▸Bear right wherever the path forks, emerging from the garden into the parking area for the museums and gardens surrounding the Music Concourse. This remarkable complex is flanked by the California Academy of Sciences (including the Steinhart Aquarium) and the striking de Young Museum. A half-domed bandstand marks the west end of the concourse, with rows of plane trees shading the fountains, statues, and benches in the plaza. The Japanese Tea Garden is off to the right (north) as you face the stage.

▸Stay to the left of the Music Concourse, passing the academy building. Walk behind the bandstand, where you will find restrooms, bike and Segway rentals, and food vendors.

▸Cross Hagiwara Tea Garden Drive to the gate to the Japanese Tea Garden. A fee is charged to tour the site. Turn left, and walk down Hagiwara Tea Garden Drive to its junction with Martin Luther King Jr. Drive.

▸Take a right onto the sidewalk that parallels Martin Luther King Jr. Drive and walk less than 100 feet to the crosswalk that leads to the Friend Gate of the San

CULTURE AND SCIENCE IN GOLDEN GATE PARK

There's so much more to Golden Gate Park than the great outdoors. A pair of San Francisco's finest cultural and scientific institutions lie near the heart of the park, on either side of the Music Concourse.

The de Young Museum houses an extensive permanent collection of fine art that encompasses most of the world's continents and nearly every artistic style and period. The de Young also brings superb traveling exhibits—featuring masters like Monet, Van Gogh, and Rembrandt—to the Bay Area. The museum, with its striking architecture, underwent an extensive remodeling following the 1989 Loma Prieta earthquake, reopening in 2005. For more information, visit deyoung.famsf.org.

The California Academy of Sciences is opposite the de Young, offering an entirely different but equally astounding visual, cultural, and scientific experience. It, like the de Young, was extensively remodeled around the turn of the twenty-first century, reopening in 2008. It houses a pair of San Francisco's most beloved longtime attractions, the Steinhart Aquarium, where visitors can immerse themselves in an underwater wonderland, and the Morrison Planetarium, devoted to interpreting the physical universe. The academy also sports a three-story rain-forest exhibit and a living roof. While arguably the focus is on educating kids, there isn't an adult who visits the academy who isn't wowed by the experience.

Another longtime attraction on the Music Concourse is the Japanese Tea Garden. Built for the 1894 California Mid-Winter Exposition, this serene garden—with its carefully crafted gates and bridge, its hills and waters based on classic rural Japanese gardens—is a great place to stop and have a cup of tea.

And just off the concourse: the San Francisco Botanical Garden. The paths that loop through what was formerly the Strybing Arboretum (rechristened in 2010) lead visitors into gardens featuring plants from around the world as well as close to home, from exhibits of flora from New Zealand, South America, and Asia to native plants of California. Other gardens focus on fragrance, the primordial, and rhododendrons. The 55-acre garden boasts more than 8,000 different plants, including magnolias that enliven the garden in winter, when other plants remain hunkered down waiting for spring. The garden also houses a small but excellent bookstore featuring a wide selection of gardening and botanical books. The Helen Crocker Russell Library of Horticulture, with its 18,000-volume collection, is open to the public. For more information about the botanical garden, call (415) 661-1316 or visit sfbotanicalgarden.org. A fee is charged to tour the gardens; it's free for San Francisco residents.

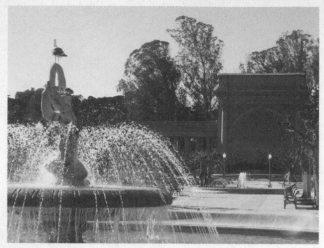
The Music Concourse in Golden Gate Park is flanked by the de Young Museum and the California Academy of Sciences.

Francisco Botanical Garden. Take a right onto the asphalt path directly opposite the gardens, heading up into a grove of trees.

▸Pass a no-longer-used exit from the Japanese Tea Garden, and veer left at the next intersection. Head uphill and away from the tea garden.

▸Climb the set of concrete stairs that leads to the edge of the roadway that encircles Stow Lake. Cross the road and turn right, following the asphalt path along the shoreline. Stow Lake draws visitors by the hundreds on weekends: picnickers, parents with strollers, kids and elders feeding the ducks, and families exploring the lake by boat.

▶Reach a paved path/road that veers left and across the concrete Roman Bridge. Cross the bridge and turn right onto the broad dirt trail that circles the base of Strawberry Hill, the little mountain that dominates the island in the middle of Stow Lake. Stay right as you circumnavigate the island; paths and stairways lead left and steeply up to the top of the hill.

▶Pass the stone Rustic Bridge, the ornate Golden Gate Pavilion (a gift to San Francisco from its sister city, Taipei, Taiwan), and the tumble of Huntington Falls as you complete the loop around Strawberry Hill.

▶Arrive back at the Roman Bridge and cross to the mainland. Turn left and walk to the Boathouse, where you will find restrooms, a snack bar, and boat, rickshaw, and bicycle rentals. Detailed maps of Golden Gate Park are available at the snack bar. The Boathouse is a great place to take a breather. You can check out the turtles sunning themselves on half-submerged logs, watch families set off to explore the lake in pedal boats, and fend off the always-hungry gulls, geese, and ducks of Stow Lake.

▶When you are ready to move on, retrace your steps along the lakeshore and return to the asphalt path that drops from the lakeside roadway to the backside of the Japanese Tea Garden.

▶Descend the concrete stairs. Turn left at the bottom of the stairs (a right will lead you back to the Friend Gate of the botanical gardens). Follow the left-hand path out to John F. Kennedy Drive.

▸At the crosswalk, cross John F. Kennedy Drive to the park's extensive Rose Garden. Depending on the time of year, you may want to stop and smell the roses.

▸Turn right and walk along the sidewalk that parallels John F. Kennedy Drive.

▸Arrive back at the Conservatory of Flowers and the end of this walk.

Walk 16: The Presidio

🌿 👫

General location: In northwestern San Francisco, just south of the Golden Gate Bridge

Special attractions: Natural and restored landscapes; historical architecture

Difficulty: Moderate; almost entirely on dirt paths

Distance: 3.1 miles

Estimated time: 1.5 hours

Services: Parking, restrooms, visitor information center. The trails are part of the Golden Gate National Recreation Area (GGNRA).

Restrictions: Not wheelchair accessible. Dogs must either be leashed or under voice control, depending on where you are walking in the GGNRA. Dog droppings must be picked up. Contact the GGNRA for the most current pet regulations.

For more information: The San Francisco Travel Association, 900 Market St., Hallidie Plaza, San Francisco, CA 94102-2804; (415) 391-2000; sanfrancisco.travel. The GGNRA Visitor Information Center for the Presidio of San Francisco is located in Building 105 on Montgomery Street, at the parade ground of the Main Post (the brick barracks closest to the bay front). The visitor center is open Thurs through Sun from 9 a.m. to 4 p.m.

Getting started: This walk begins at the corner of Sheridan Avenue and Montgomery Street on the southwest corner of the Main Post parade ground. GPS: N37 47.974' / W122 27.589'

(1) From the intersection of Market, Ninth, Hayes, and Larkin Streets near the Civic Center, veer left onto Hayes and go 3 blocks. Turn right onto Franklin Street and go about 1.75 miles to Lombard Street. Turn left onto Lombard and go 11 blocks to Broderick Street (stay in the left-hand lane). Just after Broderick, as the traffic curves to the right, remain on Lombard and follow the sign at the stoplight to the Presidio. Go 1.5 blocks on Lombard and enter the Presidio through the Lombard Gate. Turn right onto Presidio Boulevard at the first stop sign. Continue straight through several stops—you are now on Lincoln Boulevard—and pass by the foot of the main parade ground, now a large parking lot.

(2) From the Golden Gate Bridge southbound, pass through the far right tollbooth and take an immediate right at the 25th Avenue exit, onto Merchant Road. Turn left at the first stop sign onto Lincoln Boulevard and continue on Lincoln as it twists and turns through the Presidio for about 1.5 miles to the main parade ground.

There is ample parking in the large paved lot on the parade ground. A fee is charged.

Public transportation: The San Francisco Municipal Railway (Muni) provides bus service to the Presidio. Contact Muni for information about schedules, fares, and accessibility (sfmta.com, tripplanner.transit.511.org). The PresidioGo Shuttle provides service within the Presidio of San Francisco, as well as routes that link downtown to the park. Visit presidiobus.com for maps and information.

Overview: This remarkable route rambles through the blend of military history and green space that is the Presidio of San Francisco. Founded in 1776 by Spanish troops intent on colonizing the wilds of California, this outpost has changed hands three times. Little remains of what the Spanish and Mexican militaries erected on the site, but the Americans, when they acquired this prime piece of San Francisco real estate, made extensive use of the property. Its forts, batteries, hospitals, barracks, and airfield are all part of the military legacy.

Under American leadership the Presidio remained a military installation until 1994, when it passed to the National Park Service. The Presidio Trust, a federal agency charged with securing "non-federal resources to the park to ensure that it would ultimately be sustained without direct annual taxpayer support," was created shortly thereafter. The concept of a private/public partnership to sustain a national park was entirely new at the time and met with great skepticism. But as of 2013 the Presidio Trust has fulfilled its mandate, and the park's future is secure. As part of the funding plan, many of the Presidio's historic buildings—including those at Fort Mason, another former military facility now integrated into the GGNRA—house a wide variety of nonprofit organizations and for-profit businesses.

This walk begins among the historic buildings on the Presidio's Main Post and then proceeds up through a beautiful woodland. Though the forest path feels secluded, on any given day you will encounter fellow walkers, joggers, and folks on outings with their dogs. The forest used to cover much of the Presidio grounds, but as part of a restoration project some of the trees have been removed, and portions of the route wind through areas that harken back to San Francisco's early days, when the landscape was composed of sand dunes blasted by ocean winds. Drop down to El Polin Spring in Tennessee Hollow and you'll see what the restoration has revealed; the process is well established on the slopes below Inspiration Point, where native plant species of the rare serpentine grassland have been nurtured by the park and thrive.

The Presidio forest is still in evidence though, recognized as an important component of the post's identity. The forest was the result of an ambitious tree-planting project undertaken in the late nineteenth century; between 1886 and 1897 the army planted 100,000 trees (200 types) here. The project was designed, in the words of Major W. A. Jones, "to crown the ridges, border the boundary fences and cover the areas of sand and marsh waste with a forest that will generally seem continuous, and thus appear immensely larger than it really is."

Much to the benefit of present-day San Franciscans, military use of the Presidio—in one of those ironies of history—has preserved a spectacular natural area from the development that would undoubtedly have occurred on this beautifully sited and priceless real estate.

The Walk

▶Start at the corner of Sheridan Avenue and Montgomery Street, on the west side of the Presidio's main parade ground. The visitor center is located in one of five identical buildings built as enlisted men's barracks from 1895 to 1897; two of these buildings were used to hospitalize troops injured in the Philippines during the Spanish-American War. Other barracks house the offices of the Presidio Trust and the Walt Disney Family Museum.

▶Cross Sheridan and walk uphill 2 short blocks to Moraga Avenue.

▶Turn left onto Moraga and walk to Funston Avenue, passing Pershing Square on your left. The square commemorates Brigadier General John Joseph Pershing, whose wife and three children perished in a house fire on this site in 1915 while Pershing was on military duty on the Mexican border. General Pershing would go on to command the American expeditionary force in Europe during World War I. Just beyond the square, at the corner of Graham Street, stands the Spanish-style one-story building that served as the Presidio's Officers Club. A bit farther on is the post chapel, built in 1864 and modified in the 1950s.

▶At the corner of Moraga and Funston Avenue, turn right and walk around to the back of Pershing Hall (now the posh Inn at the Presidio). At the corner of Funston and Hardee Street near the inn parking lot, you'll find the signed trailhead for the Ecology Trail.

▶Head uphill on the broad, graded Ecology Trail, entering the Presidio forest. Stay left when you reach the clearing not far above the trailhead, continuing uphill into the woods.

▶Pass a gate on the left and continue uphill through the dense shade. Ignore any side trails you might encounter; the main trail is well defined, and the use of social trails is harmful to the ecosystem.

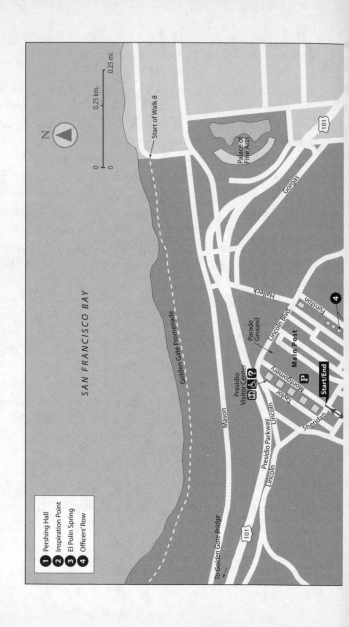

SAN FRANCISCO BAY

N

0   0.25 km.
0   0.25 mi.

Start of Walk 8

Golden Gate Promenade

Palace of Fine Arts

101

Gorgas

Halleck

Parade Ground

Mason

Lincoln Blvd

Funston

Presidio Visitor Center

Main Post

Lincoln

Presidio Parkway

Lincoln

Taylor

Montgomery

P

Start/End

Sheridan

4

To Golden Gate Bridge

101

1 Pershing Hall
2 Inspiration Point
3 El Polin Spring
4 Officers' Row

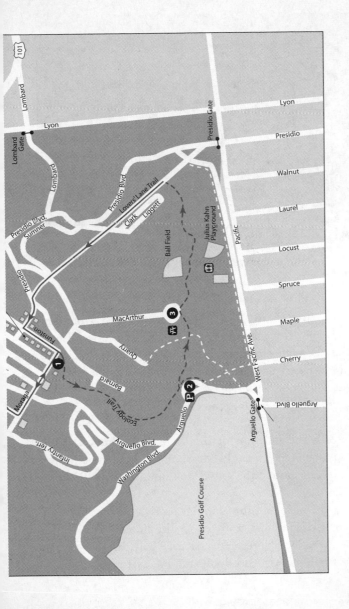

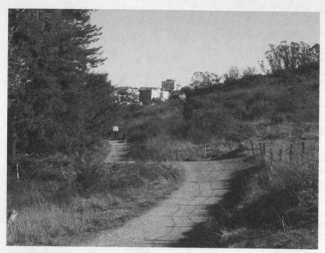

The Ecology Trail leads up through a rare, restored serpentine grassland.

▶The trail leaves the forest for the restored meadowlands below Inspiration Point. Views open of the surrounding cityscape. This restoration project involved reestablishing several endangered species, among them Presidio clarkia, Marin dwarf flax, San Francisco owl's clover, coast rock cress, and the San Francisco gum plant, which prefer the rare serpentine earth found on this hillside.

▶Reach the junction of the trails to Inspiration Point, Mountain Lake, and El Polin Spring (0.8 mile). Stay right, traversing around the hillside toward Inspiration Point.

▶At the next trail junction, go up right and uphill on a staircase, climbing 150 feet to Inspiration Point. This overlook, with interpretive signage and parking for cars that pull off Arguello Boulevard, presents sweeping views across the Presidio forest to San Francisco Bay, and of the sparkling slopes of Russian and Telegraph Hills. A historical marker at the overlook shows photographs taken from this ridge in 1880, when the dunes were bare between here and the Main Post, and in 1882, after the army had planted thousands of trees in orderly rows.

▶Retrace your steps to the second junction, where the trails to Inspiration Point, El Polin Spring, and Mountain Lake meet. Go right on the trail to El Polin Spring, descending through a stand of stately redwoods. The clearing surrounding El Polin spring floats in and out of view at the base of the hill.

▶Cross a roadway and continue down through a stand of Monterey pines.

▶The trail drops into the El Polin Spring clearing at 1.3 miles. The spring has a long history, used by the Ohlone in the days before colonization and by the Spanish after they established the presidio. Now the spring, in the Tennessee Hollow drainage, is ringed by a crushed-stone trail lined with interpretive signs. Housing for Presidio residents lies off to the left (north), and the city streets peek over the hilltop to the right (south).

▶After you've toured the restored spring area, pick up the switchbacking path that climbs out of the hollow. Go left on the signed connector to the Mountain Lake Trail, the Julius Kahn playground, and the Bay Area Ridge Trail.

RESTORING THE HABITATS OF ENDANGERED SPECIES

As you walk through the Presidio, the Marin Headlands, and other parts of the Golden Gate National Recreation Area (GGNRA), you may come upon signs marking an "Endangered Species Habitat Restoration" area.

What are these areas, and why are they so important?

It turns out that many of the plants commonly seen in the Bay Area are not native. The eucalyptus, Monterey pine, and Monterey cypress that seem so much at home in San Francisco were introduced to help break the winds that hammered the exposed headlands and cliff tops. The grasses that cloak the hillsides were inadvertently introduced by the Spanish, who imported cattle carrying nonnative seed in their hooves. Hills that once stayed green year-round now green up in winter and toast to a golden brown in summer.

Since the National Park Service acquired properties now part of the GGNRA from the US Army and other landowners, it has made habitat restoration—especially for endangered species—a top priority. Often this means removing introduced plants that have altered local ecosystems significantly enough to make them inhospitable to endangered species like the mission blue butterfly in the Marin Headlands, or rare native plants like coast rock cress or San Francisco gum plant in the Presidio. In the case of the mission blue, Monterey pines prevent the healthy survival of the butterfly's host plant, the silver lupine.

These restoration projects do not mean that the park service will remove all the trees and other nonnative plants in the Presidio. In fact, it is committed to preserving the historic forests planted here by the military and early settlers. At the same time, however, where it makes good environmental sense, park employees and volunteers continue to remove introduced species, allowing native plants—and in some cases, insects, birds, and animals—to reclaim home turf.

Walkers can help sustain these restoration efforts by staying on clearly marked trails and heeding the signs that herald the return of native species. For more information, contact the GGNRA (nps.gov/goga).

▶Circle the parking lot below the playground (which is out of sight, but you can hear the sounds of children playing), and take the first left, onto a broad sandy path that runs behind the ball field. The path climbs relatively steeply and the sand, which harkens back to the dunes of yesteryear, makes the walking a bit more difficult.

▶Ignore the unsigned path that breaks left at the 2-mile mark, staying right and continuing to climb. Just beyond you'll enter a clearing in the West Pacific Grove, where a stand of elderly Monterey cypress, with a canopy so tangled and dense it would keep you dry in a mild rain shower, was replaced with one hundred seedlings of the same species in 2009.

▶Take the path to the left out of the clearing, climbing toward Lovers' Lane.

▶Arrive on Lovers' Lane and go left, heading downhill on the paved path. Lined with lampposts and shaded by eucalyptus, Lovers' Lane is the oldest trail in San Francisco, used first by the Spanish to travel between the presidio and Mission Dolores, 3 miles away, and later by off-duty officers leaving to visit civilian San Francisco—and often their sweethearts, hence the name. The trail descends past a line of brick houses built in the 1930s that once housed the families of enlisted men.

▶Cross Liggett Avenue (2.3 miles) and continue downhill on Lovers' Lane.

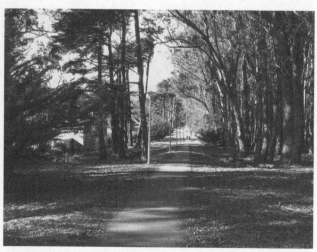

A walk down Lover's Lane in the Presidio retraces the steps of Spanish soldiers traveling to Mission Dolores.

▸At the bottom of the hill, cross MacArthur Avenue, continue over a small brick footbridge, and then climb for a short block to the intersection where Barnard Avenue dead-ends into Presidio Boulevard. Cross Presidio at the crosswalk and continue straight for 1 block, along Presidio, to Funston Avenue. Four large homes built in the 1880s as officers' residences flank this block, fine examples of Queen Anne and Stick-style architecture.

▸Cross Funston and turn left. At this point—where Presidio intersects Funston—you are passing the original entrance to the Spanish-era Presidio.

▸Walk uphill on Funston for 1 block along Officers' Row. Built in 1862, these homes are the oldest still standing in the Presidio. The simple three- or four-bedroom wooden structures housed officers who had previously shared six rooms in an adobe building left by the Spanish.

▸Turn right at Moraga and walk 5 blocks to Montgomery.

▸Turn right onto Montgomery and walk back to Sheridan and the end of this walk.

Walk 17: Wolf Ridge Loop in the Marin Headlands

General location: On the Marin Headlands, directly across the Golden Gate Bridge from San Francisco

Special attractions: Historical landmarks; spectacular views of San Francisco, the Marin Headlands, Mount Tamalpais, and the Pacific Ocean; wildlife viewing and bird watching

Difficulty: Strenuous, with some long uphill stretches. The trail surface, both paved and dirt, is often uneven.

Distance: 6.5 miles

Estimated time: 3.5 hours

Services: Restrooms, picnic sites, water, visitor information center

Restrictions: Not wheelchair accessible. The Coastal Trail section of this walk is subject to continual erosion and the National Park Service reroutes the trail as necessary. Watch for clearly marked detours. You won't find shade along this route; bring a hat and plenty of water. Be careful on cliffs and at the beach; staying on the trail will keep you free of eroding cliff edges and sneaker waves. Each year the park service rescues a number of people who fall off cliffs or get swept away by heavy surf or riptides. Dogs must either be leashed or under voice control. In some areas pets are prohibited entirely to protect sensitive resources. Dog droppings must be picked up. Contact the Golden Gate National Recreation Area (GGNRA) for the most current pet regulations.

For more information: Golden Gate National Recreation Area, Fort Mason, Building 201, San Francisco, CA 94123-0022; (415) 561-4700; nps.gov/goga. The Marin Headlands Visitor Center is in the Fort Barry Chapel at the intersection of Field and Bunker Roads near Rodeo Lagoon; (415) 331-1540; nps.gov/goga/marin-headlands .htm; open daily from 9:30 a.m. to 4:30 p.m.

Getting started: This walk begins in the parking lot at the far end of Fort Cronkhite in the Marin Headlands. GPS: N37 49.937' / W122 32.336'

(1) From the intersection of Market, Ninth, Hayes, and Larkin Streets near the Civic Center, veer left onto Hayes and go 3 blocks. Turn right onto Franklin Street and go approximately 1.75 miles to Lombard Street. Turn left onto Lombard and continue 3 miles, following the signs to the Golden Gate Bridge. Immediately after crossing the bridge, take the Alexander Avenue exit. Turn left at the first stop, go under the freeway, and then turn right onto Conzelman Road, following the signs for the GGNRA and Marin Headlands. After climbing steeply into the headlands for 1.5 miles—the views are spectacular—turn right onto McCullough Road and head downhill, away from the ocean. Turn left onto Bunker Road and head west, passing the Marin Headlands Visitor Center in the Fort Barry chapel. Continue on Bunker Road, past Rodeo Lagoon and the buildings of Fort Cronkhite, to the road's end, where you'll find a large parking lot and the trailhead.

(2) If you are driving to the headlands from the San Francisco Peninsula, you can avoid downtown San Francisco by taking I-280 north to the 19th Avenue / Park Presidio exit just beyond Daly City (stay in the left lanes on the freeway). Continue on CA 1 north—on Junipero

Serra Boulevard, 19th Avenue, and Park Presidio—to the Golden Gate Bridge. On the north side of the bridge take the Alexander Avenue exit. Turn left at the first stop, go under the freeway, and then turn right onto Conzelman Road, following the signs for the GGNRA and Marin Headlands. After climbing steeply for 1.5 miles, turn right onto McCullough Road, and head downhill to the junction with Bunker Road. Turn left onto Bunker Road and head west, past Rodeo Lagoon, to the road's end, a large parking lot, and the trailhead.

(3) From Marin County drive on US 101 south, taking the Sausalito exit (just before the Golden Gate Bridge). Turn left at the first stop, then immediately right onto Conzelman Road, following the signs for the GGNRA and Marin Headlands. After climbing steeply into the headlands for 1.5 miles, turn right onto McCullough Road and head downhill to the junction with Bunker Road. Turn left onto Bunker Road and continue past Rodeo Lagoon to the parking lot and trailhead.

Public transportation: Bus 76X of the San Francisco Municipal Railway (Muni) runs to Fort Cronkhite on Sat and Sun and some holidays. It is wheelchair accessible. Contact Muni for information about schedules, fares, and accessibility (sfmta.com, tripplanner.transit.511.org).

Overview: Stark and blessed with stunning vistas, the Marin Headlands are rich in human history and natural beauty. This vigorous walk—okay, let's call it what it is: a hike—takes you past remnants of the area's military past to overlooks with breathtaking panoramic views, through a landscape both wild and accessible.

Be prepared to work on this route, which climbs 880 feet to gain the top of Wolf Ridge before dropping back down to the ocean. The walk links four separate trails into a pleasing loop: the Coastal Trail, the Wolf Ridge Trail, the Miwok Trail, and the portion of the Rodeo Lagoon Loop, which runs alongside Bunker Road.

Start by climbing away from Fort Cronkhite, one of many US Army facilities turned over to the National Park Service as the GGNRA came into being. The fort overlooks Rodeo Beach, and amenities include picnic areas (the grills are wheelchair accessible), restrooms, and water. Though the surf looks sketchy and uninviting to swimmers, you're likely to share the beach with surfers hardy enough to risk the savage undertows.

The rolling coastal hills and dramatic seaside cliffs of the headlands have been home to army gun emplacements since the mid-nineteenth century, and it was only with the introduction of long-range missiles that the batteries on the headlands became obsolete. The ruins of these batteries dot the climb.

Although military tunnels have been blasted into the hillsides and the cattle that once grazed on these hills decimated the native grasses, the headlands remain rich habitat for many varieties of plants and animals. A distinctive coastal scrub, made up of a mix of such plants as California sagebrush, California blackberry, coyote bush, sticky monkeyflower, currant, and the ubiquitous poison oak, covers these hillsides. Common wildflowers include California poppies, Douglas iris, blue dick, rock cress, lupine, and columbine. You will almost certainly see small lizards darting across the trail, and lucky walkers may catch glimpses of deer, foxes, and bobcats. Birds frequently seen in the headlands include western grebes, cormorants, herons, turkey vultures, gulls, great horned owls, scrub jays, and even the rare brown pelican. Hawk Hill, also known as Battery 129, is nearby, where birders gather in flocks during spring and fall migrations to observe and count the raptors that soar overhead.

As you climb into the headlands, do not forget to look behind you, back to the lovely curve of Rodeo Beach and, across the water, to the Golden Gate Bridge and the city of San Francisco, luminous in sunlight or shrouded in fog.

Note: This route can be combined with the trail around Rodeo Lagoon (Walk 18). When you reach trail's end alongside Bunker Road, instead of turning right, turn left and walk to the guardrail alongside the roadway. Descend the short set of stairs, and follow the narrow dirt track past the Marin Headlands Visitor Center and along the southern rim of the lagoon, emerging on Rodeo Beach within view of the parking lot and the start of this walk.

The Walk

▸Start at the western end of the parking lot at Fort Cronkhite. Pass through a gate and onto the old asphalt road that leads up into the hills. At the sign turn left onto the Coastal Trail (labeled Hikers Route), which climbs onto the hillside. You'll double-back on this trail to take the right-hand trail/road (signed Bikers Route) to reach Battery Townsend and beyond.

▸Informal trails intersect the main route; stay left, walking along the edge of the continent and enjoying spectacular views of the Pacific.

▸Pass through a gate (0.7 mile).

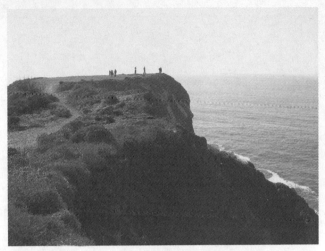

The overlook at Tennessee Point offers endless views across the Pacific.

▶Follow the trail out through a bower of Monterey pine to a large overlook on a flat-topped bluff on Tennessee Point. When you've taken in the views, return as you came to the junction of the hike/bike routes. The social trails that lead up into the hills toward Battery Townsend may be tempting, but they are not maintained and using them damages the habitat.

▶Back at the junction, turn left onto the bikers route portion of the Coastal Trail (1.4 miles).

▶Follow the paved road up to Battery Townsley. To explore the site, walk through the tunnel out to the emplacement for gun #1, a massive hollow in the hillside with unimpeded views of the Golden Gate (2 miles).

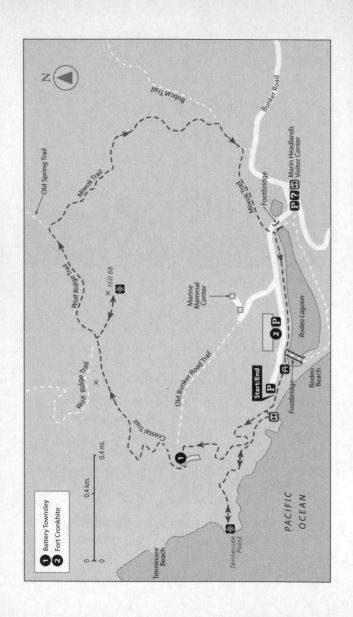

N

Old Spring Trail

Bobcat Trail

Miwok Trail

Bunker Road

Miwok Trail

Footbridge

Marin Headlands
Visitor Center

P ?

Wolf Ridge Trail

× *Hill 88*

Marine Mammal
Center

Rodeo Lagoon

2 P

Wolf Ridge Trail

×

Start/End

P

Footbridge

Old Bunker Road Trail

Rodeo
Beach

Coastal Trail

1

PACIFIC
OCEAN

Tennessee Point

Tennessee Beach

0   0.4 km.

0   0.4 mi.

1 Battery Townsley
2 Fort Cronkhite

▸Return to the trail and continue on the signed Coastal Trail, which climbs the first of several sets of stairs. The road dropping to the right, Old Bunker Road, heads down to the Marine Mammal Center, located above Fort Cronkhite.

▸As you ascend, look back (south) to catch increasingly spectacular views of Fort Cronkhite, Rodeo Beach, the Pacific, and the city of San Francisco itself. Among the San Francisco sights visible on clearer days are Sutro Tower and Twin Peaks, the forested hills of Lands End, and the sandy expanse of Ocean Beach. The bleating of the foghorns and banging of buoy bells rise from the water, mingling with the cries of the hawks that circle overhead.

▸Pass through a saddle. The trail intersects the paved road just beyond. Follow the paved road uphill to the right to the next sign for the Coastal Trail.

▸Take the Coastal Trail (a set of stairs) up and to the left. Do not follow the road; a landslide has taken it out a few curves ahead.

▸Reach the top of the staircase and continue to the right on the signed Coastal Trail.

▸At the next junction, with a barrier, stay right on the signed Coastal Trail (3.5 miles). You are back on pavement at this point, which you will follow to the top of Hill 88.

▸Pass the junction with the Wolf Ridge Trail (on the left), which you will return to after you've finished the ascent

EXPLORING THE HEADLANDS

The routes that climb Wolf Ridge and circle Rodeo Lagoon are spectacular, but the Marin Headlands offer so much more to those with the time and desire to explore. Here is a sampling.

- Point Bonita Lighthouse: Open on a limited basis, the historic lighthouse, moved to its perch on the edge of the continent in 1876, is reached via a 125-foot-long tunnel carved through the hillside by Chinese immigrants and a pedestrian suspension bridge spanning a cleft in the rocky shoreline that churns with breaking surf.
- The Golden Gate Overlook at Battery Spencer: A short walk leads through the ruins of a battery to a broad concrete apron that offers iconic views of the Golden Gate Bridge and the San Francisco skyline.
- Tennessee Cove: This crescent of sand cupped between steep bluffs lies at the end of one of the most pleasant trails in the headlands. The Tennessee Valley Trail is mostly flat and wanders through a riparian zone thick with reeds and willow before passing a tiny lagoon and spilling onto the beach.
- Kirby Cove: This one's a local favorite. Follow a broad track downhill from Conzelman Road to a tiny, protected cove

backed by the ruins of Battery Kirby and facing the Golden Gate, with the bridge and the maritime traffic that passes beneath—tankers, sailboats, ferries, and the occasional kayak—in full view.

- Hawk Hill: A short climb through Battery 129 leads to one of the premier raptor-viewing sites on the Pacific Flyway.
- Nike Missile Site: Not a hike but not to be missed. In their last incarnation, the fortifications at the Marin Headlands were outfitted for the Cold War. At the Nike Missile Site, one of eleven such sites in the Bay Area, artifacts of the nuclear age are preserved and, more spectacularly, on display. You can tour the facility, which is open to the public Thurs, Fri, and Sat from 12:30 to 3:30 p.m. (call the Marin Headlands Visitor Center at 415-331-1540 for details).

More information about these sites and trails, as well as other points of interest in the headlands, is available at nps.gov/goga.

to the top of Hill 88. Follow the paved road uphill to the right, toward the gate.

▶You'll have attained the high point of this hike at the 3.8-mile mark, on the summit of Hill 88. The hill is topped with the ruins of a military radar station built during the early 1950s. This "ghost" station is a wonderful spot for a picnic lunch and offers some of the best views on this walk.

▸Retrace your steps down the roadway to the turnoff for Wolf Ridge Trail. Turn right and begin descending the dirt Wolf Ridge Trail, which circles around the backside of Hill 88.

▸Wolf Ridge Trail descends steeply, carrying you into a cooler, moister, shadier microclimate. Watch your step and watch your speed, as this section of trail is extremely steep. Keep an eye out for songbirds in the bushes, snakes and lizards sunning themselves on rocks (or the treadway), and perhaps a bobcat or black-tailed deer. Off to the left, you can look down onto the Tennessee Valley Trail and, farther off, the houses of Mill Valley scattered among the trees. Mount Tamalpais, known locally as the Sleeping Lady, dominates the northern skyline, dressed in a thick green gown of oak and bay laurel.

▸At the bottom of the steep descent, the trail levels out and even climbs a bit before a final descent to the signed junction with the Miwok Trail at 4.9 miles.

▸Turn right onto the Miwok Trail and continue to descend. You'll share this broad dirt track with mountain bikers, and enjoy views down into the expansive Gerbode Valley.

▸As you near the base of the Miwok Trail, Bunker Road and the buildings of Fort Cronkhite come into view.

▶At the junction with the Bobcat Trail, which leads into Gerbode Valley, stay right on the Miwok Trail (6 miles). The Miwok Trail passes a marshy area on the left and ends beside an old warehouse on Bunker Road. Straight across the road lie the vivid green waters of Rodeo Lagoon.

▶Cross Bunker Road and, turning right, walk on the trail alongside the lagoon. This trail will take you back to Fort Cronkhite and the end of this walk.

Walk 18: Rodeo Lagoon

🍃 👫 📷

General location: On the Marin Headlands, across the Golden Gate Bridge from San Francisco

Special attractions: Beach and lagoon with shorebird and seabird viewing; Marine Mammal Center; views of the Marin Headlands and the Pacific Ocean

Difficulty: Easy, with a brief stretch of deep sand on Rodeo Beach

Distance: 1.5 miles

Estimated time: 1 hour

Services: Restrooms, water, picnic sites, visitor information center

Restrictions: Not wheelchair accessible, but beach wheelchairs can be used on portions of the route. Contact the GGNRA at (415) 561-4700 a week in advance of your visit to reserve a chair. Be careful on cliffs or at Rodeo Beach; heed signs warning of dangerous surf. Each year the National Park Service rescues a number of people who fall off cliffs or get swept away by heavy surf or riptides. Dogs must either be leashed or under voice control. In some areas pets are prohibited entirely to protect sensitive resources. Dog droppings must be picked up. Contact the Golden Gate National Recreation Area (GGNRA) for the most current pet regulations. Mountain bikes are not allowed on this trail, although they are allowed elsewhere in the Marin Headlands. Swimming, fishing, and boating are forbidden in Rodeo Lagoon.

For more information: Golden Gate National Recreation Area, Fort Mason, Building 201, San Francisco, CA

94123-0022; (415) 561-4700; nps.gov/goga. The Marin Headlands Visitor Center is in the Fort Barry Chapel at the intersection of Field and Bunker Roads near Rodeo Lagoon; (415) 331-1540; nps.gov/goga/marin-headlands .htm; open daily from 9:30 a.m. to 4:30 p.m.

Getting started: This walk begins in the parking lot at the far end of Fort Cronkhite in the Marin Headlands. GPS: N37 49.937' / W122 32.336'

(1) From the intersection of Market, Ninth, Hayes, and Larkin Streets near the Civic Center, veer left onto Hayes and go 3 blocks. Turn right onto Franklin Street and go approximately 1./5 miles to Lombard Street. Turn left onto Lombard and continue 3 miles, following the signs to the Golden Gate Bridge. Immediately after crossing the bridge, take the Alexander Avenue exit. Turn left at the first stop, go under the freeway, and then turn right onto Conzelman Road, following the signs for the GGNRA and Marin Headlands. After climbing steeply into the headlands for 1.5 miles—the views are spectacular—turn right onto McCullough Road and head downhill, away from the ocean. Turn left onto Bunker Road and follow it past the Marin Headlands Visitor Center, Rodeo Lagoon and the buildings of Fort Cronkhite, to the road's end, where you'll find a large parking lot and the trailhead.

(2) If you are driving to the headlands from the San Francisco Peninsula, you can avoid downtown San Francisco by taking I-280 north to the 19th Avenue / Park Presidio exit just beyond Daly City (stay in the left lanes on the freeway). Continue on CA 1 north—on Junipero Serra Boulevard, 19th Avenue, and Park Presidio—to the Golden Gate Bridge. On the north side of the bridge, take the Alexander Avenue exit. Turn left at the first stop, go

under the freeway, and then turn right onto Conzelman Road, following the signs for the GGNRA and Marin Headlands. After climbing steeply for 1.5 miles, turn right onto McCullough Road, and head downhill to the junction with Bunker Road. Turn left onto Bunker Road and head west, past Rodeo Lagoon, to the road's end, a large parking lot, and the trailhead.

(3) From Marin County, drive south on US 101, taking the Sausalito exit (just before the Golden Gate Bridge). Then turn left at the first stop, then immediately right onto Conzelman Road, following signs for the GGNRA and Marin Headlands. After climbing steeply for 1.5 miles, turn right onto McCullough Road and head downhill to the junction with Bunker Road. Turn left onto Bunker Road and continue past Rodeo Lagoon to the road's end at the parking lot and trailhead.

Public transportation: Bus 76X of the San Francisco Municipal Railway (Muni) runs to Fort Cronkhite on Sat and Sun and some holidays. It is wheelchair accessible. Contact Muni for information about schedules, fares, and accessibility (sfmta.com, tripplanner.transit.511.org).

Overview: The loop around Rodeo Lagoon is short, but it offers many pleasures, especially for birders. With its brevity, lack of challenging hills, and stretch of sandy beach, this walk is ideal for families with young children.

The walk begins inauspiciously, wedged between the shoreline of Rodeo Lagoon and Bunker Road. But the setting is still evocative, with the sound of surf crashing onto Rodeo Beach behind, and the red roofs of Fort Cronkhite splashing color onto the greens, grays, and blues of the surroundings. In winter powerful waves cross the beach and enter the lagoon, an annual infusion of salt water that

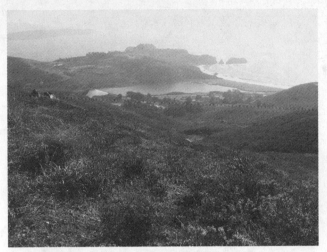
Rodeo Lagoon shimmers in the late afternoon sun.

creates ideal habitat for salt-tolerant plants and animals. As the ocean subsides with the arrival of spring, it leaves behind enough sand to reestablish the beach, re-creating the separation between lagoon and ocean once more.

Though the lagoon is stagnant much of the year, the water provides rich nutrients for tiny aquatic animals and plants that thrive here, which in turn attract all manner of hungry waterfowl—from snowy egrets to many varieties of ducks and the rare brown pelican. These pelicans, once endangered, can be found on the lagoon during spring, summer, and fall. Salamanders mate here, and you can sometimes see raccoons, foxes, and other mammals in the dense brush along the shore.

Take your time as you circle Rodeo Lagoon. This brief but lovely walk also provides access to the Marin Headlands Visitor Center, where you can visit educational exhibits,

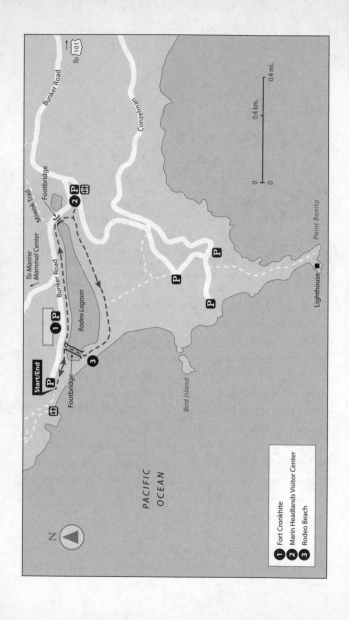

PACIFIC
OCEAN

N

To 101

Bunker Road

Conzelman

0   0.4 km.
0   0.4 mi.

Footbridge

Miwok Trail

2 P ♿

To Marine
Mammal Center

Bunker Road

Start/End

P

1 P

♿

Footbridge

Rodeo Lagoon

3

Bird Island

P

P

P

Point Bonita

Lighthouse ■

1 Fort Cronkhite
2 Marin Headlands Visitor Center
3 Rodeo Beach

purchase gifts, and meet with staff who can answer almost any question about the headlands.

Note: This walk may be combined with the longer hike onto Wolf Ridge (Walk 17). The two routes meet in the Fort Cronkhite parking lot; once you've looped around the lagoon, you can head up the hill to the overlook at Tennessee Point or travel all the way to the summit of Hill 88 and back.

The Walk

▶Start in the parking lot at the far end of Fort Cronkhite. Exit the parking lot, cross Bunker Road, and turn left, following the path alongside the roadway and passing a wooden footbridge that leads to Rodeo Beach. Check out the interpretive panels that describe the wildlife of the lagoon and the natural forces that shape the lagoon and beach each year.

▶Continue down the roadside path, climbing gently to cross the street leading left and up to the Marine Mammal Center. You might be able to hear the cries of the seals and sea lions in residence and recovery at the center as you pass.

▶The roadside path descends gently alongside the reeds and rushes that line the lagoon.

▶Reach the crosswalk/junction with the end of the Miwok Trail, at the point where Bunker Road turns sharply right toward the Marin Headlands Visitor Center (0.5 mile).

THE MARINE MAMMAL CENTER

The mission of the Marine Mammal Center, located just up the hill off Bunker Road in Fort Cronkhite, "is to expand knowledge about marine mammals—their health and that of their ocean environment—and to inspire their global conservation." To that end, the organization rescues and rehabilitates ill, injured, and abandoned marine mammals in its hospital—it has treated more than 18,000 since 1975. Its education programs, which may involve slide shows, artifacts, or excursions along the coast, have reached thousands of schoolchildren and their parents and teachers, helping them better understand the whales, dolphins, otters, seals, and sea lions that the center serves. And the center's important science program conducts studies of the threats—both from disease and environmental changes—that these marine mammals face.

As a nonprofit organization, the Marine Mammal Center depends upon memberships, donations, and volunteers to achieve its mission. Find out how to help at marinemammalcenter.org or by calling (415) 289-7325. You can also visit and tour the center. It is open daily from 10 a.m. to 5 p.m., and admission is free.

Turn right with the path, crossing the levy at the east end of the lagoon.

▶At the signed junction of the Lagoon and Coastal Trails, go right and downhill on the Lagoon Trail, diving into dense riparian brush.

▶Cross a footbridge and climb stairs to a second trail junction. The Marin Headlands Visitor Center, housed in the old Fort Barry Chapel, is on the right. To continue the loop, go left on the Lagoon Trail.

▶Follow the shoreline path, now more secluded, passing under bowers of eucalyptus and enjoying spectacular views of the still waters. Pause and watch: You are likely to see mallards, pelicans, cormorants, great blue herons, snowy egrets, a variety of songbirds, and a host of other seabirds and shorebirds on the open water, in the shallows, or flitting through the brush on the shoreline. Binoculars or a camera will help.

▶Climb a short hill, then descend to the beach (1.3 miles). Trail's end is visible across the expanse of sand: Pick a line and make your crossing. The walking is easier closer to the surf line, where water packs the sand. In addition to gazing out over the Pacific, you can also watch black-clad surfers catching waves just offshore. If you stay on the lagoon side of the beach, you'll hitch up with the footbridge you passed near the start of the hike, which will deposit you back onto Bunker Road.

▶Climb the sand bank alongside Bunker Road and arrive back at the trailhead.

Appendix A: Other Sights

San Francisco and the surrounding region offer an almost infinite array of attractions. Those listed below are just a sampling of what you can enjoy in the greater Bay Area. Not all involve walking, but each has delighted millions of tourists and residents. Have a great time.

In San Francisco
Cable Car Barn and Museum
1201 Mason St.
(415) 474-1887
cablecarmuseum.org
This wonderful museum—set in the still-operating cable car powerhouse, or winding house—takes you through the history of San Francisco's legendary cable car system. Its excellent exhibits are well worth the visit, but it is the viewing area downstairs—where you can watch the great wheels wind the cables—that truly fascinates most visitors.

Mission Dolores (Mission San Francisco de Asis)
Dolores and 16th Streets (3321 16th St.)
(415) 621-8203
missiondolores.org
San Francisco's oldest structure—the mission was established in 1776 and built in 1782—Mission Dolores is a monument to the city's Spanish founders and the influence of Catholic missions in early California. After surviving several major earthquakes, the 1906 fire, and two centuries of use, this modest mission, with its gorgeous reredos and poignant garden, remains an important part of the Mission District, to which it lends its name.

San Francisco Zoo
Sloat Boulevard at the Great Highway
(415) 753-7080
sfzoo.org
The San Francisco Zoo features the Doelger Primate Discovery Center, where you can watch rare and endangered apes and monkeys in environments that simulate their natural habitats. More than 1,000 species make their home at the zoo, including Australian koalas, seldom seen in this country. Interactive and computer exhibits are among the educational attractions, as is a mini-zoo designed specifically for kids.

Outside San Francisco
Alcatraz Island
San Francisco Bay
(415) 561-4900
nps.gov/alcatraz
Home for many years to a federal prison, this island is one of the most frequently visited places in the Golden Gate National Recreation Area. Besides touring the cellhouse, you can also see the first lighthouse on the West Coast; walk along the island's cliffs, enjoying unimpeded views of San Francisco, the bay, and passing ships; and learn more about the natural history of this austere and intriguing place. To reach Alcatraz from San Francisco, take a Blue & Gold ferry from Pier 41. Blue & Gold ferries also provide transport to Angel Island State Park, which was used during World War II as a Japanese internment center and is a wonderful place to take a hike (angelisland.org).

Bay Area Discovery Museum
East Fort Baker; 557 McReynolds Rd., Sausalito
(415) 339-3900
baykidsmuseum.org
This kid-oriented museum uses hands-on exhibits to depict the Bay Area's rich human and natural history. It is a perfect place to spend an afternoon with the family. While at East Fort Baker, you can also check out the fishing pier and abandoned gun batteries, take a pleasant walk near Horseshoe Bay, or just enjoy the sunny weather on this side of the bay.

Muir Woods National Monument
Mill Valley
(415) 388-2595
nps.gov/muwo
Named for John Muir, the father of modern conservation and champion of Yosemite National Park and the Sierra Nevada, Marin County's Muir Woods preserves a grand remnant of the virgin redwood forests that once flourished in much of the Bay Area. The hiking trails in Muir Woods range from an easy 2-mile meander along paved paths among the giants to a thigh-pumping 8.5-mile climb onto the hills overlooking Point Reyes and the Pacific. This extremely popular piece of the Golden Gate National Recreation Area is very crowded on summer weekends; you'll likely have to park on the highway outside the monument and ride the shuttle down to the site.

Point Reyes National Seashore
Point Reyes Station
(415) 464-5100
nps.gov/pore
For walkers who want to explore the wild side of the San Francisco Bay Area, this absolutely gorgeous oceanfront park 40 miles north of the city features 32,000 acres of coastal wilderness, with about 150 miles of trails. At Point Reyes you can also visit an 1860s dairy ranch, see a herd of tule elk, walk along dramatic beaches, drop down a precipitous staircase to a historic lighthouse, and take an interpretive walk along a trail that explores the rupture caused by the 1906 earthquake.

The Wine Country
In the valleys of Napa, Sonoma, Mendocino, and Lake Counties, north of San Francisco, you can explore California's famous vineyards. This region, overflowing with boutique wineries and fabulous restaurants, is a bacchanalian pleasure ground. Not only can you sip world-class vintages, but you can tour scenic back roads, enjoy spectacular river valleys, walk along the ocean, hike through redwoods, and climb into oak woodlands. Set yourself up in one of the region's lovely bed-and-breakfasts and enjoy the countryside.

Appendix B: Contact Information

San Francisco Travel Association, Visitor Information Center, 900 Market St., Hallidie Plaza (at Market and Powell Streets, next to the cable car turnaround), San Francisco, CA 94102-2804; (415) 391-2000; sanfrancisco .travel. Business office: One Front Street, Suite 2900, San Francisco, CA 94111; (415) 974-6900. The San Francisco Travel Association can provide a wealth of information about San Francisco and the Bay Area.

The *San Francisco Chronicle*'s Web portal, sfgate.com, is a great source for the latest world, local, sports, and entertainment news, as well as a treasure trove of articles on good eats, recreational opportunities, and special events in San Francisco and surrounding communities.

Activities, Attractions, and Museums
Asian Art Museum of San Francisco, 200 Larkin St., San Francisco, CA 94102; (415) 581-3500; asianart.org
California Academy of Sciences (including the Steinhart Aquarium and Morrison Planetarium), 55 Music Concourse Dr., Golden Gate Park, San Francisco, CA 94118; (415) 379-8000; calacademy.org
California Historical Society, 678 Mission St., San Francisco, CA 94105; (415) 357-1848; calhist.org
California Palace of the Legion of Honor, Lincoln Park, 100 34th Ave. (34th Avenue and Clement Street), San Francisco, CA 94121; (415) 750-3600; legionof honor.famsf.org
The Cannery, 2801 Leavenworth St., San Francisco, CA 94133

Chinese Culture Center, 750 Kearny St., Third Floor, San Francisco, CA 94108; (415) 986-1822; c-c-c.org

Chinese Historical Society of America, 965 Clay St., San Francisco, CA 94108; (415) 391-1188; chsa.org

City Lights Booksellers and Publishers, 261 Columbus Ave., San Francisco, CA 94133; (415) 362-8193; city lights.com

Coit Tower, 1 Telegraph Hill Blvd., San Francisco, CA 94133; (415) 249-0995

de Young Museum, 50 Hagiwara Tea Garden Dr. (on the Music Concourse in Golden Gate Park), San Francisco, CA 94118; (415) 750-3600; deyoung.famsf.org

Embarcadero Center, (415) 772-0700; embarcadero center.com

The Exploratorium, Pier 15, San Francisco, CA 94111; (415) 528-4444; exploratorium.edu

Galería de la Raza, 2857 24th St., San Francisco, CA 94110; (415) 826-8009; galeriadelaraza.org

Ghirardelli Square, 900 North Point St., San Francisco, CA 94109; (415) 775-5500; ghirardellisq.com

Gulf of the Farallones National Marine Sanctuary Visitor Center, Old Coast Guard Station, Golden Gate Promenade, 991 Marine Dr., The Presidio, San Francisco, CA 94129; (415) 561-6622; farallones.noaa.gov

Haas-Lilienthal House, 2007 Franklin St., San Francisco, CA 94109; (415) 441-3000; sfheritage.org/ haas-lilienthal-house

Marine Mammal Center, 2000 Bunker Rd., Fort Cronkhite, Sausalito, CA 94965-2619; (415) 289-7325; marinemammalcenter.org

The Mexican Museum, Fort Mason Center, 2 Marina Blvd., Building D, San Francisco, CA 94123; (415)

202-9700; mexicanmuseum.org. The museum is slated to open in a new building in Yerba Buena Gardens in 2018.

Musée Mécanique, Pier 45 on Fisherman's Wharf, San Francisco, CA 94133; (415) 346-2000; museemecaniquesf.com

Museo Italo Americano, Fort Mason Center, 2 Marina Blvd., Building C, San Francisco, CA 94123; (415) 673-2200; museoitaloamericano.org

National Japanese American Historical Society, 1684 Post St., San Francisco, CA 94115; (415) 921-5007; njahs.org

Octagon House, 2645 Gough St., San Francisco, CA 94123; (415) 441-7512; nscda.org/museums2/ca-octagon house.html

PIER 39, Beach Street and The Embarcadero, San Francisco, CA 94133; (415) 981-7437; pier39.com

Precita Eyes Mural Arts and Visitor Center, 2981 24th St., San Francisco, CA 94110; (415) 285-2287; precita eyes.org

San Francisco Art Institute, 800 Chestnut St., San Francisco, CA 94133; (415) 771-7020; sfai.edu

San Francisco Camera Obscura and Holograph Gallery, 1096 Point Lobos Ave., San Francisco, CA 94121; (415) 750-0415; giantcamera.com

San Francisco Museum of Modern Art, 151 Third St., San Francisco, CA 94103; (415) 357-4000; sfmoma.org

USS *Pampanito,* Pier 45, Fisherman's Wharf, San Francisco, CA 94133; (415) 775-1943; maritime.org/pamp home.shtml

Yerba Buena Center for the Arts, 701 Mission St. (at Third Street), San Francisco, CA 94103-3138; (415) 978-ARTS (2787); ybca.org

Public Beaches, Gardens, and Parks
Cliff House, 1090 Point Lobos Ave., San Francisco, CA 94121; (415) 386-3330; cliffhouse.com
Fort Mason Center, 2 Marina Blvd., Building A, San Francisco, CA 94123; (415) 345-7500; fortmason.org
Fort Point National Historic Site, (415) 556-1693; nps .gov/fopo
Golden Gate National Recreation Area, Fort Mason, Building 201, San Francisco, CA 94123-0022; (415) 561-4700; nps.gov/goga
Golden Gate Park, McLaren Lodge, San Francisco, CA 94117; golden-gate-park.com
Japanese Tea Garden, 75 Hagiwara Tea Garden Dr., San Francisco, CA 94118; japaneseteagardensf.com
Lands End Lookout, 680 Point Lobos Ave.; San Francisco, CA 94121; (415) 426-5240; nps.gov/goga/plan yourvisit/landsend.htm
Marin Headlands Visitor Information Center, Fort Barry Chapel at the intersection of Field and Bunker Roads; (415) 331-1540; nps.gov/goga/marin-headlands .htm
Presidio of San Francisco Visitor Information Center, Building 105, Montgomery Street, Main Post, San Francisco, CA 94123; (415) 561-4323; nps.gov/prsf
San Francisco Botanical Garden, 1199 9th Ave., San Francisco, CA 94122; (415) 661-1316; sfbotanical garden.org

Other San Francisco City Parks
Hyde Street Pier, foot of Hyde Street; San Francisco, CA 94109; (415) 561-7000

San Francisco Maritime Museum, 900 Beach St., San Francisco, CA 94109; (415) 561-7000

San Francisco Maritime National Historical Park, Aquatic Park to Hyde Street Pier, San Francisco, CA 94109; (415) 561-7000; www.nps.gov/safr

San Francisco Recreation and Parks Department, McLaren Lodge, 501 Stanyan St., San Francisco, CA 94117; (415) 831-2700; sfrecpark.org. The San Francisco Recreation and Parks Department oversees hundreds of parks, recreation centers, swimming pools, public works of art, and stairways.

Hotels

To find lodging that suits your tastes and pocketbook, check with the San Francisco Travel Association (sanfrancisco .travel/stay) or visit any of the popular online travel outlets (Expedia, Orbitz, Hotels.com).

Word of mouth is still the best way to find a great place to stay. The list below includes a handful of excellent hotels, including a few of the downtown classics and several smaller "boutique" hostelries with plenty of character.

Hotel Beresford, 635 Sutter St.; (415) 673-9900; beresford.com

Clift San Francisco, 495 Geary St.; (415) 775-4700; morganshotelgroup.com/originals/originals-clift -san-francisco

The Fairmont San Francisco Hotel, 950 Mason St.; (415) 772-5000; fairmont.com/san-francisco

Grand Hyatt San Francisco Hotel, 345 Stockton St.; (415) 398-1234; grandsanfrancisco.hyatt.com

Hotel Bohème, 444 Columbus Ave.; (415) 433-9111; hotelboheme.com

Hotel Rex, 562 Sutter St.; (415) 433-4434; jdvhotels
.com/hotels/california/san-francisco-hotels/hotel-rex
Hotel Triton, 342 Grant Ave.; (415) 394-0500; hotel
triton.com
Hyatt Regency San Francisco, 5 Embarcadero Center;
(415) 788-1234; sanfranciscoregency.hyatt.com/en/hotel/
home.html
InterContinental Mark Hopkins San Francisco, 999
California St.; (415) 392-3434; intercontinentalmark
hopkins.com
The San Remo Hotel, 2237 Mason St.; (415) 776-8688;
sanremohotel.com
Stanford Court, 905 California St.; (415) 989-3500;
stanfordcourt.com
Tuscan Inn, 425 North Point; (415) 561-1100; tuscan
inn.com
Westin St. Francis Hotel, 335 Powell St.; (415) 397-
7000; westinstfrancis.com

Transportation
AC Transit: Transbay Temporary Terminal, First and
Mission Streets; dial 511, then say "AC Transit" for
the AC Transit menu, then say, "Customer Relations";
actransit.org
Amtrak: (800) USA-RAIL (872-7245) (for reservations
and schedule information); amtrak.com
Bay Area Rail Transportation (BART): PO Box 12688,
Oakland, CA 94604-2688; (415) 989-2278; bart.gov
Blue & Gold Fleet: Ferry service from PIER 39 / Pier
41 at Fisherman's Wharf to Alameda/Oakland, Alcatraz,
Angel Island, Sausalito, Tiburon, and Vallejo; (415) 705-
8200; blueandgoldfleet.com

Caltrain: 1250 San Carlos Ave., San Carlos, CA 94070-1306; (800) 660-4287, (650) 508-6448 TTY; caltrain.com

Golden Gate Ferry: Providing service from the Golden Gate Ferry Terminal at the Ferry Building on the Embarcadero at the foot of Market Street to Sausalito and Larkspur; dial 511 in the Bay Area, (415) 455-2000 outside the Bay Area; goldengate.org; 511.org

Golden Gate Transit: PO Box 9000, Presidio Station, San Francisco, CA 94129-0601; dial 511 in the Bay Area, (415) 455-2000 outside the Bay Area; goldengate.org or 511.org

SamTrans: 1250 San Carlos Ave., PO Box 3006, San Carlos, CA 94070-1306; (800) 660-4287, (650) 508-6448 TTY; samtrans.com

San Francisco Municipal Railway (Muni): 949 Presidio Ave., San Francisco, CA 94115; 11 South Van Ness Ave., San Francisco, CA 94103 (customer service center); (415) 673-MUNI; sfmta.com

SFBay 511: A comprehensive travel-planning service for the Bay Area; dial 511; 511.org

Appendix C: Great Tastes

San Francisco—together with the fertile countryside that surrounds it—is one of America's food meccas. The city is home to one of the greatest concentrations of restaurants per capita in the nation. The following list includes just a few of the fine restaurants, cafes, and coffeehouses found along the walks in this guide, along with a few other favorites. If you are interested in surveying the full range of eateries to be found in the Bay Area, pick up a local newspaper or ask around: The person sitting next to you on the bus bench no doubt has a special place to share.

Beach Chalet Brewery & Restaurant, 1000 Great Hwy., San Francisco; (415) 386-8439; beachchalet.com. Great casual food and beer brewed on the premises. Spectacular views of the ocean.

Betelnut, 2030 Union St., San Francisco; (415) 929-8855; betelnutrestaurant.com. Serving small and large plates of pan-Asian cuisine.

Blue Barn, 2237 Polk St., San Francisco (and other locations); (415) 655-9438; bluebarngourmet.com. Salads and sandwiches incorporating locally sourced ingredients that are fully customizable.

Buena Vista Cafe, 2765 Hyde St., San Francisco; (415) 474-5044; thebuenavista.com. This landmark bar-cafe is the home of the original Irish coffee in America. Also famous for its breakfasts and its Ramos fizzes.

Cafe Bastille, 22 Belden Place, San Francisco; (415) 986-5673; cafebastille.com. A classic but casual French cafe with outside tables located downtown.

Cafe Claude, 7 Claude Ln., San Francisco; (415) 392-3505; cafeclaude.com. A French cafe on a charming narrow street featuring wine, hors d'oeuvres, and daily specials. Jazz nightly.

Cafe de la Presse, 352 Grant Ave., San Francisco; (415) 398-2680; cafedelapresse.com. A bit of Paris with outdoor seating on a busy street.

Cafe deStijl, 1 Union St., San Francisco; (415) 291-0808; destijl.com. This cafe near the Embarcadero is a tribute to Dutch modernist architecture.

Caffe Greco, 423 Columbus Ave., San Francisco; (415) 397-6261; caffegreco.com. Outstanding among the many North Beach coffeehouses.

Caffe Trieste, 601 Vallejo St., San Francisco; (415) 392-6739; caffetrieste.com. Still a quintessential North Beach gathering spot for artists and writers.

Capps Corner, 1600 Powell St., San Francisco; (415) 989-2589; cappscorner.com. Full and hearty Italian multicourse meals served family-style in a lively, old-time atmosphere.

Cooks and Company, Fort Mason Center, San Francisco; (415) 673-4137; fortmason.org/residents/directory. Cooks and Company is a great place to pick up a quick snack or a lunch before setting out along the Marina Green.

E&O Asian Kitchen, 314 Sutter St., San Francisco; (415) 693-0303; eosanfrancisco.com. Pacific Rim cuisine.

Firefly Restaurant, 4288 24th St., San Francisco; (415) 821-7652; fireflyrestaurant.com. This arty Noe Valley gathering place gets great reviews for its imaginative and subtle dishes.

Fog City, 1300 Battery St., San Francisco; (415) 982-2000; fogcitysf.com. A diner gone fancy near the Embarcadero and Levi's Plaza.

Fresca Nouveau Peruvian Cuisine, 3945 24th St., San Francisco (and other locations); (415) 695-0549; frescasf .com/noe-valley. A Noe Valley hot spot.

Greens Restaurant, Fort Mason Center, Building A, San Francisco; (415) 771-6222; greensrestaurant.com. Vegetarian cuisine par excellence. Spacious with gorgeous views of the bay.

Henry's Hunan Restaurant, 924 Sansome St., San Francisco; (415) 956-7727; henryshunanrestaurant.com. Hot and spicy cuisine from Hunan Province. High quality for many years; now with additional locations in the city. Great for large groups.

House of Nanking, 919 Kearny St., San Francisco; (415) 421-1429; houseofnanking.net. This storefront cafe at the edge of Chinatown is always crowded, but it's worth the wait. Always fresh ingredients and inexpensive.

Il Fornaio, 1265 Battery St., San Francisco; (415) 986-0100; ilfornaio.com. This casually elegant restaurant offers everything from pizza and pasta to full Italian meals.

Isobune Sushi, 1737 Post St., San Francisco; (415) 563-1030; isobunesushi.com. Located in the heart of Japantown, the sushi (served in boats) will delight families.

Kuleto's, 221 Powell St., San Francisco; (415) 397-7720; kuletos.com. This downtown standout sports a busy, sophisticated atmosphere and imaginative, delicious pasta. Reservations recommended.

Legion of Honor Cafe and Garden Terrace, California Palace of the Legion of Honor, Lincoln Park (34th Avenue and Clement Street), San Francisco; (415) 750-3595; legionofhonor.famsf.org/legion/visiting/legion-honor-caf. Snacks and beverages to fuel your museum explorations.

Liguria Bakery, 1700 Stockton St., San Francisco; (415) 421-3786. The Liguria sells only focaccia—the very best.

Lovejoy's Tea Room, 1351 Church St., San Francisco; (415) 648-5895; lovejoystearoom.com. Absolutely charming and a favorite with kids.

Mario's Bohemian Cigar Store Cafe, 566 Columbus Ave., San Francisco; (415) 362-0536. A landmark meeting place for North Beach locals.

Marnee Thai Restaurant, 2225 Irving St. (plus a location on Ninth Avenue), San Francisco; (415) 665-9500; marneethaisf.com. Serving great Thai cuisine since 1986.

Restaurant LuLu, 816 Folsom St., San Francisco; (415) 495-5775; restaurantlulu.com. South of Market not far from Yerba Buena Gardens. LuLu has a spectacular interior, extraordinary food (with a wood-fired oven and rotisserie), friendly service, and reasonable prices.

Rose Pistola, 532 Columbus Ave., San Francisco; (415) 399-0499; rosepistolasf.com. One of San Francisco's hottest restaurants. Features innovative Northern Italian cuisine.

Sutro's at the Cliff House, 1090 Point Lobos Ave., San Francisco; (415) 386-3330; cliffhouse.com/sutro. The greatest ocean views from every table, plus the Terrace Room, with the greatest ocean views from every bar stool.

Swensen's Ice Cream, Union and Hyde (1999 Hyde St.), San Francisco; (415) 775-6818; swensens.com. The original store of a well-known chain. The fabulous ice cream is made right here.

Tadich Grill, 240 California St., San Francisco; (415) 391-1849; tadichgrill.com. Founded in 1849, this Financial District tradition is known for its seafood and its crowds.

Tosca Cafe, 242 Columbus Ave., San Francisco; (415) 986-9651; toscacafesf.com. A North Beach joint famous for its long bar, film celebrity clientele, and brandy-laced cappuccinos.

Vesuvio Cafe, 255 Columbus Ave., San Francisco; (415) 362-3370; vesuvio.com. More a bar than a cafe, Vesuvio is a relic of the Beat era in North Beach.

Waterfront Restaurant, Pier 7, San Francisco; (415) 391-2696; waterfrontsf.com. This beautiful restaurant sits right on the bay.

Yukol Place Thai Cuisine, 2380 Lombard St., San Francisco; (415) 922-1599; www.yukolthai.com. Great food, quiet atmosphere, and soothing on your wallet as well.

Yum Yum Fish, 2181 Irving St., San Francisco; (415) 566-6433; yumyumfishsushi.com. Located in the Sunset District near Golden Gate Park. There are a few tables, but Yum Yum sells most of its sushi and sashimi to go. Great stop on the way to a picnic in the park or at the beach.

Zuni Cafe, 1658 Market St., San Francisco; (415) 552-2522; zunicafe.com. A downtown favorite that highlights seasonal ingredients.

Appendix D: Useful Phone Numbers and Websites

The area code for San Francisco is 415.

San Francisco Police Department: Emergency 911; nonemergency (415) 553-0123, (415) 626-4357 TTY; sf-police.org

San Francisco City & County Sheriff's Department: Emergency 911; nonemergency (415) 554-7225; sfsheriff.com

San Francisco Fire Department: Emergency 911; (415) 558-3200 (information); sf-fire.org

San Francisco General Hospital: (415) 206-8000; sfdph.org

San Francisco Department of Public Health: (415) 206-8000; sfdph.org

National Park Police: (415) 561-5505 (San Francisco Field Office)

San Francisco Public Library (Main Branch): (415) 557-4400 (general Information); sfpl.org

Road and Weather Conditions: Dial 511; 511.org

San Francisco Chronicle: (415) 777-1111; sfchronicle.com

San Francisco Examiner: (415) 359-2661; sfexaminer.com

California State Highway Patrol: Emergency 911; nonemergency (800) 835-5247; chp.ca.gov

For general information about city services, dial 311 (415-701-2311 outside San Francisco).

Appendix E: Books and Films

San Francisco is the subject of scores of guidebooks and travelogues, and as the West Coast's unrivaled literary center, the city on the bay has spawned countless novels, screenplays, and poems. The following bibliography is only a beginning. You will find many more books about this incredible city in its friendly bookstores, museum shops, and visitor centers. And remember that San Francisco has served as the setting for more than one hundred feature films.

Fiction

Berriault, Gina. *Women in Their Beds: New and Selected Stories.* Washington, DC: Counterpoint, 1997. A collection of thirty-five "jewel-box perfect" stories by an exceptional Bay Area writer.

Hammett, Dashiell. *The Maltese Falcon.* New York: Vintage Crime/Black Lizard, 1992. Featuring Sam Spade, this atmospheric masterpiece of suspense fiction is set in the San Francisco of the 1920s.

Kingston, Maxine Hong. *Tripmaster Monkey: His Fake Book.* New York: Vintage International, 1990. The story of a free-spirited Chinese-American writer in San Francisco during the late 1960s.

Maupin, Armistead. *Tales of the City.* New York: Harper Perennial Library, 1994. Made into a miniseries for public television, this wise and funny novel—originally serialized in the San Francisco Chronicle—captures the magic and romance of Maupin's chosen city during the 1970s.

Norris, Frank. *McTeague: A Story of San Francisco.* New York: New American Library, 1997. This gritty realist novel depicts San Francisco at the turn of the twentieth century.

Tan, Amy. *The Joy Luck Club.* New York: Ivy Books, 1994. A rich and involving novel set in San Francisco that recounts the interwoven stories of four Chinese immigrant mothers and their daughters.

Twain, Mark. *Roughing It.* New York: New American Library, 1994. Partly fact and partly tall tale, this is Twain's colorful account of his early adulthood in Nevada, San Francisco (and elsewhere in California), and Hawaii.

Nonfiction

Brechin, Gray. *Imperial San Francisco: Urban Power, Earthly Ruin.* Berkeley: University of California Press: 1999; 2006. A compelling analysis of the men and forces that propelled San Francisco to the forefront of cultural and political California.

Bronson, William. *The Earth Shook, the Sky Burned.* San Francisco: Chronicle Books, 1986. This extensively illustrated history captures the excitement and trauma of the 1906 earthquake and fire.

Chinn, Thomas W. *Bridging the Pacific: San Francisco Chinatown and Its People.* San Francisco: Chinese Historical Society of America, 1989. This thoroughly researched study gives you Chinatown's inside story.

Delehanty, Randolph. *San Francisco: The Ultimate Guide.* San Francisco: Chronicle Books, 1995. Delehanty is the dean of San Francisco guidebook authors, and this is the most complete guide to the City by the Bay.

Gustaitis, Rasa, and Jerry Emory. *San Francisco Bay Shoreline Guide.* Berkeley: University of California Press, 1995. A superb guide to the natural and manmade wonders of the bay shoreline.

Herron, Don. *The Dashiell Hammett Tour.* San Francisco: City Lights Books, 1991. The definitive guide to novelist Hammett's—and his legendary detective Sam Spade's—San Francisco.

Richards, Rand. *Historic San Francisco: A Concise History and Guide.* San Francisco: Heritage House, 1991. Includes not only a readable history of the city but a series of fascinating tours organized around that history.

Unterman, Patricia. *Patricia Unterman's Food Lover's Guide to San Francisco.* San Francisco: Chronicle Books, 1997. An essential guide to San Francisco's astonishing culinary offerings.

Wach, Bonnie. *San Francisco As You Like It: 20 Tailor-Made Tours for Culture Vultures, Shopaholics, Java Junkies, Fitness Freaks, Savvy Natives, and Everyone Else.* San Francisco: Chronicle Books, 1998. A fun and eclectic guide to San Francisco's attractions.

Woodbridge, Sally, and John Woodbridge. *San Francisco Architecture.* San Francisco: Chronicle Books, 1992. A thorough and useful guide to the city's built environment.

Films

Barbary Coast (1935); *Birdman of Alcatraz* (1962); *Bullitt* (1968); *The Conversation* (1974); *Dark Passage* (1947);

Dirty Harry (1971); *Escape from Alcatraz* (1979); *Flower Drum Song* (1961); *The Joy Luck Club* (1993); *The Lady from Shanghai* (1948); *The Maltese Falcon* (1941); *Mrs. Doubtfire* (1993); *Pacific Heights* (1990); *The Presidio* (1988); *San Francisco* (1936); *Sister Act* (1990); *Towering Inferno* (1974); *Until the End of the World* (1991); *Vertigo* (1958)

San Francisco Place Names

To get a basic history lesson based on place names in San Francisco, check out sfstreets.noahveltman.com, an inter-active place-name map generated by Noah Veltman, a Knight-Mozilla OpenNews Fellow at the BBC.

Appendix F: Local Walking Clubs and Tours

Walking Clubs
Bay Bandits Volksmarch Club

The Bay Bandits Volksmarch Club is part of the American Volkssport Association, a network of clubs that sponsor noncompetitive walking, swimming, and biking events. Events are posted at the California Volkssport Association (cva4u.org). To receive a free general information packet that explains volkssporting and the American Volkssport Association, call the AVA at (800) 830-WALK or visit ava.org.

San Francisco Walking Tours
San Francisco City Guides
(415) 557-4266
sfcityguides.org
Features free tours throughout the city led by well-informed volunteers.

Foundation for San Francisco's Architectural Heritage
(415) 441-3000
sfheritage.org
Explore the city's architecturally significant neighborhoods.

Javawalk
(415) 673-9255
javawalk.com
Offers a 2-hour caffeine tour of North Beach, Chinatown, and Union Square.

San Francisco Mural Walks
Precita Eyes Mural Arts Center
(415) 285-2287
precitaeyes.org
Leads you past the Mission District's eighty-plus murals.

San Francisco Strolls
(415) 297-6534
strollsanfrancisco.com
Features thirty-three walks customized to the character of each distinctive neighborhood explored.

Walk San Francisco
(415) 431-WALK
walksf.org
This pedestrian advocacy group also hosts walking events.

Index

About the Authors

Liz Gans grew up in the San Francisco Bay Area and spent many years in San Francisco working as marketing director for Banana Republic and Gap. Since moving to Montana, she has directed a visual arts museum, designed databases, and worked as a management consultant. She is president of Zadig LLC and loves to walk the hills of San Francisco.

Rick Newby, a former editorial director at Falcon Publishing, is a poet, essayist, and editor. His previous guidebooks include *Great Escapes: Montana State Parks* (Falcon, 1989), and he edited—with Suzanne Hunger—the collection of essays *Writing Montana: Literature under the Big Sky* (1996). A convert to the pleasures of walking San Francisco, Newby is a veteran walker. He is the author of a book of poems entitled *Old Friends Walking in the Mountains.*

Tracy Salcedo-Chourré has written guidebooks to a number of destinations in California and Colorado, including *Best Hikes Near Reno-Lake Tahoe, Hiking Lassen Volcanic National Park, Best Hikes Near Sacramento, Best Rail-Trails California, Exploring California's Missions and Presidios, Exploring Point Reyes National Seashore and the Golden Gate National Recreation Area,* and Best Easy Day Hikes guides to San Francisco's Peninsula, North Bay, and East Bay, San Jose, Lake Tahoe, Reno, Sacramento, Fresno, Boulder, Denver, and Aspen. She lives with her family in California's Wine Country. You can learn more by visiting her website at laughingwaterink.com.